Department
of
Economic
and
Social
Affairs

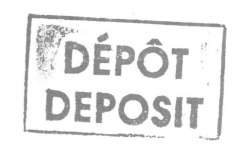

World *YOUTH* Report
2005

Young people today, and in 2015

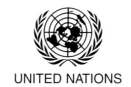

UNITED NATIONS

DESA

The Department of Economic and Social Affairs of the United Nations Secretariat is a vital interface between global policies in the economic, social and environmental spheres and national action. The Department works in three main interlinked areas: (i) it compiles, generates and analyzes a wide range of economic, social and environmental data and information on which States Members of the United Nations draw to review common problems and to take stock of policy options; (ii) it facilitates the negotiations of Member States in many intergovernmental bodies on joint courses of action to address ongoing
or emerging global challenges; and (iii) it advises interested Governments on the ways and means of translating policy frameworks developed in United Nations conferences and summits into programmes at the country level and, through techncal assistance, helps build national capacities.

UN2
ST/ESA/301

ST/ESA/301
ISBN 92-1-130244-7

United Nations publication -
Sales No. E. 05 IV.6
05 44737 - 3,000

Foreword

Young people today, and in 2015

Young people hold the key to society's future. Their ambitions, goals and aspirations for peace, security, development and human rights are often in accord with those of society as a whole. The international development agenda is centred around the achievement of the eight Millennium Development Goals (MDGs) incorporated in the United Nations Millennium Declaration. Each of these Goals relates directly or indirectly to the well-being of children and young people.

We are living in a very youthful world, indeed, with almost half of the current global population under the age of 25. There are 1.2 billion young people in the world today, and the next generation of youth (children presently below the age of 15) will be half again as large, numbering 1.8 billion. Thanks to the global consensus that led to the adoption of the MDGs, young people are increasingly becoming the focus of international attention.

With over 200 million youth living in poverty, 130 million illiterate, 88 million unemployed, and 10 million living with HIV/AIDS, the case for investing in young people today is clear. However, world leaders must also commit themselves to ensuring the well-being of the next generation; today's children will be the youth of 2015-the year targeted for the achievement of many of the MDGs. In 2003, a quarter of all children in the developing world were malnourished. Eleven million children under the age of five die each year, mostly from preventable and treatable diseases; if this trend continues, 110 million of the world's youngest children will have perished before the current group of five-year olds reaches the threshold age of youth in 2015. Moreover, 115 million children are currently not in school. These statistics suggest that the young people of 2015 will face enormous challenges unless a much greater effort is made to achieve the MDG targets set for that year.

The MDGs relevant to the current generation highlight youth employment, maternal health, and reduced exposure to HIV/AIDS and other preventable diseases. For the future generation of youth, the MDGs address universal primary education, reductions in child mortality, and improved maternal health. This indicates that the MDGs are in many respects "youth development goals".

The year 2005 marks not only the five-year review of the implementation of the United Nations Millennium Declaration and of progress in achieving the MDGs, but also the tenth anniversary of the World Programme of Action for Youth to the Year 2000 and Beyond, adopted by the General Assembly in 1995. Predating the Millennium Declaration by several years, this Programme of Action constituted the first global blueprint for effective national youth policies. Highlighting ten priority areas of youth policy in a practical, comprehensive policy plan, it has served as an essential reference point for many Governments all over the world.

A number of important changes have taken place since the adoption of the World Programme of Action for Youth. Young people, more than any other age group, have been adversely affected by developments relating to globalization, the ageing of society, rapid advances in information and communication technology, the HIV/AIDS epidemic, and armed conflict. The direct relevance of these areas of concern to the lives of young people was recognized in the adoption of General Assembly resolution 58/133 of 2003 and further validated by their inclusion in the World Youth Report, 2003, which provided an extensive evaluation of what had been achieved both in these five areas and in the original ten areas of policy priority identified in the World Programme of Action for Youth.

This second edition of the World Youth Report reflects a very different approach from that of the earlier edition. The main findings of the 2003 Report remain valid. In the present publication, the 15 areas of priority are grouped into three clusters that reflect a somewhat broader focus on youth in a global economy, youth in civil society, and youth at risk. To provide a better understanding of the realities faced by the current generation of young people, each of the three sections of the Report focuses on a particular cluster and includes a brief review of all the priorities it encompasses, as well as a more detailed examination and analysis of one topic of particular relevance. The topic highlighted in part I is poverty among young people in its various dimensions. Before the 2003 Report was published, little was known about the numbers of young people living in poverty, let alone the dynamics characterizing their unique circumstances and experiences in this context. Part II zooms into some of the dramatic changes occurring in relation to young people's social and cultural development. While there is still enormous diversity among young people worldwide, the processes of urbanization and globalization and rapid advances in information and communication technology have arguably contributed to the emergence of a new global media-driven youth culture. These trends have each had an impact on young people's socialization and on youth activism and other forms of civic engagement. Part III of the Report highlights the impact of conflict on young people. While most youth manage to make the transition from childhood to adulthood in a safe and peaceful environment, large numbers of young people are not so fortunate; the past 15 years have witnessed enormous growth in domestic and international armed conflict.

Too often, youth policies are shaped by negative stereotypes of young people, with excessive attention given to delinquency, drug abuse and violence. This type of policy focus ignores the majority of youth, who do not engage in such high-risk behaviours, and diverts attention away from the need for structural investments in education, health care and employment creation.

Investing in youth starts with investing in children. Strengthening policy and resource commitments now with the aim of achieving the relevant MDG targets in the coming decade will produce enormous benefits for the young people of 2015. Today's young people will also benefit from efforts in this regard, and as they have demonstrated repeatedly, they are partners in working towards these global development goals. Too many young people continue to live in dire circumstances; there is no time to lose in scaling up investments in our planet's youngest residents.

It is my sincere hope that with the five-year review of progress towards achieving the MDGs and the tenth anniversary of the World Programme of Action for Youth, and through publications such as this one, world leaders will recognize the youth of today as untapped resources for development and peace.

José Antonio Ocampo
Under-Secretary-General

Acknowledgements

This *Report* was produced through the collaboration of United Nations staff, experts and young people.

The core team consisted of Fred Doulton, Charlotte van Hees, Julie Larsen, Sylvie Pailler, Joop Theunissen and Mike Thiedke, the staff of the United Nations Programme on Youth, Division for Social Policy and Development, Department of Economic and Social Affairs. Drafts of the Report were reviewed by Bob Huber, Sergei Zelenev and Johan Schölvinck of the Division for Social Policy and Development. The following experts contributed individual chapters to the publication: Richard Curtain, consultant, Melbourne (chapter 2); Karen Moore, Child Poverty Research Centre and Institute for Development Policy and Management, University of Manchester (chapter 3); David Buckingham, University of Newcastle, and Tommi Hoikkala, Finnish Youth Research Network, Helsinki (chapter 5); Ronald Kassimir, Social Science Research Council, New York (chapter 6); and Jane Lowicki-Zucca, consultant, New York (chapter 8).

Consultations held at various meetings and workshops contributed to the preparation of this Report. Part I benefited from discussions at the Regional Workshop on Youth in Poverty in Southeast Asia, hosted by the Government of Indonesia in Yogyakarta in August 2004. Parts II and III are based on presentations made during workshops held at United Nations Headquarters in April 2004 and May 2005 respectively.

We would like to thank the young people who represented their organizations at the various consultations held in preparation for the ten-year review of the World Programme of Action for Youth to the Year 2000 and Beyond, in particular those who attended the consultative meetings in Coimbra, Portugal, and in New York in January and February 2005, as well as those who contributed to a review meeting organized by the Agence Intergouvernementale de la Francophonie (AIF) and held in Cairo in May 2005.

We would also like to acknowledge the contributions made to the conceptual framework of this Report, in particular the valuable input provided by our colleagues at the United Nations Children's Fund, United Nations Educational, Scientific and Cultural Organization, United Nations Environment Programme, United Nations Human Settlements Programme, United Nations Population Fund,

Office of the United Nations High Commissioner for Refugees, United Nations Office on Drugs and Crime, International Labour Organization, Food and Agriculture Organization of the United Nations, World Bank, United Nations Millennium Campaign, Youth Employment Network, Economic Commission for Africa, Economic Commission for Europe, Economic Commission for Latin America and the Caribbean, Economic and Social Commission for Asia and the Pacific, Economic and Social Commission for Western Asia, and United Nations Volunteers, as well as by various intergovernmental organizations, including AIF, the Commonwealth Youth Programme, and the Council of Europe.

We wish to express particular gratitude to the Governments of Indonesia and Portugal for graciously hosting the events that contributed to the preparation of the Report. The working papers and presentations for these events are available at www.un.org/youth > Our work > Meetings and Workshops.

Finally we wish to acknowledge the editor Ms Terri Lore, the design and layout team of Diana de Filippi and Nancy Watt Rosenfeld. ●

Photo credits:
From the exhibition 'Chasing the Dream, youth faces of the Millennium Development Goals' (www.chasingdream.org):
—Diego Goldberg/PixelPress/UNFPA: cover, table of contents and pages 10, 19, 26, 33, 37, 42, 46, 59, 67, 68, 77, 78, 83, 90, 93, 100, 105, 106, 112, 128, 129, 132, 134, 137, 138, 142, 154 and 162.
—Anonymous/PixelPress/UNFPA: page 14.
—Michael/PixelPress/UNFPA: pages 80 and 144.

Ken Paprocki Photography: pages 9, 17, 22, 44, 51, 62, 65, 116, 127, 131, 139, 165, 171 and 181.

Rida Abboud: pages 87 and 99.

United Nations photo library: pages 31, 38, 73, 110, 119, 124, 151, 156, 161, 174, 177 and 187.

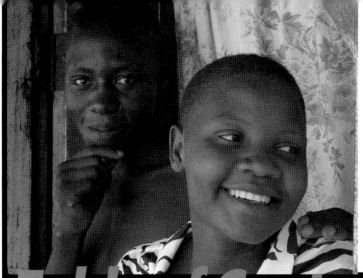

Table of Contents

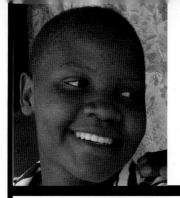

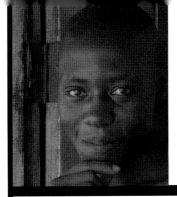

TABLES, FIGURES AND BOXES

Technical Note

In this publication, unless otherwise indicated, the term "youth" refers to all those between the ages of 15 and 24, as reflected in the World Programme of Action for Youth to the Year 2000 and Beyond. The term "young people" may be used interchangeably with the word "youth" in the text.

LIST OF ABBREVIATIONS

AIDS	acquired immune deficiency syndrome
CAFF	children associated (or formerly associated) with fighting forces
CAP	consolidated appeals process
CD	compact disc
CD-ROM	compact disc - read-only memory
DDR	(Programme on) Disarmament, Demobilization and Reintegration
DHS	Demographic and Health Survey
e-	electronic (examples include e-mail and e-commerce)
FAO	Food and Agriculture Organization of the United Nations
FGM	female genital mutilation
HIV	human immunodeficiency virus
IASC	Inter-Agency Standing Committee
ICT	information and communication technology
IDP	internally displaced person(s)
ILO	International Labour Organization
KLA	Kosovo Liberation Army
MDG	Millennium Development Goal
MONUC	United Nations Mission in the Democratic Republic of the Congo
MSEE	Minimum Standards for Education in Emergencies, Chronic Crises and Early Reconstruction
MTV	Music Television
NGO	non-governmental organization
OIOS	United Nations Office of Internal Oversight Services
OSRSGCAC	Office of the Special Representative of the Secretary-General for Children and Armed Conflict
PC	personal computer
PRSP	Poverty Reduction Strategy Paper
RHRC	Reproductive Health Response in Conflict Consortium
RUF	Revolutionary United Front (Sierra Leone)
STI	sexually transmitted infection
UNDP	United Nations Development Programme
UNEP	United Nations Environment Programme
UNESCO	United Nations Educational, Scientific and Cultural Organization
UNHCR	Office of the United Nations High Commissioner for Refugees
UNICEF	United Nations Children's Fund
VCR	video cassette recorder
WAFF	women associated (or formerly associated) with fighting forces
YEN	Youth Employment Network
YMC	Youth Media Council

INTRODUCTION
Why This Book?

For at least the past 40 years, the General Assembly of the United Nations has had a tradition of using the start of another decade of its existence to draw attention to the future leaders of the world: young people. At its twentieth session in 1965, the General Assembly adopted the Declaration on the Promotion among Youth of the Ideals of Peace, Mutual Respect and Understanding between Peoples. In 1975, it issued guidelines on three basic themes in the field of youth: participation, development and peace. The General Assembly proclaimed 1985 International Youth Year as it celebrated its fortieth anniversary, and ten years later, it agreed on the first global blueprint for youth policy: the World Programme of Action for Youth to the Year 2000 and Beyond.

As many generations of young people have come and gone, and as each decade has witnessed the emergence of a new cohort of young people between the ages of 15 and 24, youth issues have remained a prime concern for many policymakers. Many of the basic aspects of the transitional phase of life known as youth have remained the same; education, health, entry into the world of work, family formation, and productive and responsible citizenship are still among the highest priorities for young people. The Millennium Development Goals (MDGs) represent a renewed commitment to ensuring that these basic requirements are met so that young people may realize their innate potential.

It is also true, however, that the world in which young people are now making their transition into adulthood is quite different from that of ten years ago. Few foresaw the enormous impact that rapid globalization, the spread of HIV/AIDS, the explosive growth of information and communication technology (ICT), and other recent developments would have on young people's daily lives. Some of the previous generations of youth lived in a period of global ideological polarization. Gradually, they began to demand greater participation in the institutions influencing their socialization (notably the systems of education in their societies) and in democratic decision-making processes. While the latter has become a crucial element of successful youth policies worldwide, the former ideological focus has largely vanished and appears to have been replaced by new ideological conflicts.

This type of historical perspective serves to remind youth policymakers of a simple but often ignored fact: young people today are different from any of the previous generations of youth. It is essential to ensure that youth interventions are relevant and valid for the current young generation in society and not mired in the realities of times past.

MAIN FINDINGS: A SNAPSHOT OF YOUTH WORLDWIDE

This publication builds upon the *World Youth Report, 2003*. The earlier *Report* provided a detailed analysis of the ten areas of policy priority addressed in the World Programme of Action for Youth to the Year 2000 and Beyond, adopted by the General Assembly in 1995, as well as the five additional areas of concern formally acknowledged by the General Assembly in 2003 (see the list below).

The ten priority areas of the World Programme of Action for Youth to the Year 2000 and Beyond, adopted by the General Assembly in its resolution 50/81 of 1995, include the following:

1. **Education**

2. **Employment**

3. **Hunger and poverty**

4. **Health**

5. **Environment**

6	**Drug abuse**
7	**Juvenile delinquency**
8	**Leisure-time activities**
9	**Girls and young women**
10	**Youth participation in decision-making**

Five additional priority areas identified by the General Assembly in its resolution 58/133 of 2003 are as follows:

1	**Globalization**
2	**Information and communication technology**
3	**HIV/AIDS**
4	**Youth and armed conflict**
5	**Intergenerational relations**

It was decided that providing a comprehensive update on the same priority areas only two years after the issuance of the 2003 *Report* was unlikely to offer much new insight, as the global situation of young people has not changed dramatically in most respects. Nonetheless, it is appropriate to mark the tenth anniversary of the World Programme of Action for Youth with a review of major developments and the progress achieved in each of the areas of concern. Some of the main findings of the analysis are summarized in the following:

- *Poverty.* Estimates based on available poverty data from 2002 indicate that some 209 million young people, or 18 per cent of all youth, live on less than US$ 1 per day, and 515 million live on less than US$ 2 per day. As poverty indicators are usually not disaggregated by age, it is unclear whether the poverty situation of young people has improved or deteriorated since 1995. The effects of intergenerational transfers on young people's income and well-being also need to be better understood.

- *Education.* Since 1995, the number of children completing primary school has continued to increase, and four out of five young people in the eligible age group are now in secondary school. Tertiary enrolment has risen as well; it is estimated that some 100 million youth are presently engaged in university-level studies worldwide. The current generation of youth is the best-educated so far. However, 113 million children are not in school, and 130 million young people are illiterate.

- *Employment.* In spite of the progress achieved in education, global youth unemployment has increased to a record high of 88 million. Rates of unemployment among young people are highest in Western Asia, North Africa and sub-Saharan Africa. There is growing pressure on young people to compete in an increasingly globalized labour market.

- *Health.* Globally, young people are reaching adolescence earlier and marrying later. Premarital sexual relations appear to be increasing. Although early pregnancy has declined in many countries, it is still a major concern. HIV/AIDS is the primary cause of mortality among youth, followed by violence and injuries.

- *Environment.* Young people continue to be concerned about a sustainable future. There is a need to increase their involvement in decision-making processes that relate to the environment.

- *Leisure.* The past decade has seen growing recognition of the vital role leisure time can play in the lives of young people in terms of promoting social inclusion, access to opportunities, and overall development. Young people are increasingly seeking and finding new ways to spend their free time, both out of necessity and out of choice.

- *Drug abuse.* There has been an unprecedented increase in the use of synthetic drugs worldwide, mostly in recreational settings. The demand for illicit substances among youth in developing countries has risen to levels typically found in industrialized countries.

- *Juvenile delinquency.* Delinquency among young people perpetuates negative stereotypes and is often perceived as a threat to society. Some countries respond to this threat by imposing policies of incarceration and active deterrence, while various United Nations instruments promote social rather than judicial approaches to dealing with young offenders.

- *Girls and young women.* There has been greater awareness of gender issues among Governments. However, equal access to higher education and labour markets remains a concern in some countries. Negative stereotypes of women persist in both old and new media.

- *Participation in decision-making.* Over the past decade there has been growing recognition of the importance of youth participation in decision-making. New efforts to include young people in decision-making must take into account the significant changes occurring in the patterns and structures of youth movements.

- *Globalization.* Young people are adaptable and perhaps best able to make use of the new opportunities offered by globalization. However, large numbers of young people have not benefited from this process, especially in developing countries. Globalization has had an impact on youth employment opportunities and migration patterns, and has led to profound changes in youth culture and consumerism and in global youth citizenship and activism.

- *Information and communication technology.* The proliferation of ICT within the context of globalization over the past decade has presented both opportunities and challenges for young people. The global digital divide affects individuals of all ages, including youth.

- *HIV/AIDS.* Ten million young people, most of them in Africa and Asia, are currently living with HIV/AIDS. The epidemic has had a devastating impact on the sexual and reproductive health of young people, as they are particularly vulnerable to infection.

- *Youth and conflict.* A disproportionate number of young people have been involved in conflicts over the past decade. While an international legal framework is in place to protect minors and prevent their engagement in conflict situations, there has been no improvement on the ground.

- *Intergenerational relations.* The share of young people in the world's total population is gradually declining, and youth development will increasingly be geared towards the potential benefits it can bring to other generations. Despite its changing structure, the family remains the primary social institution for the congregation and interaction of generations.

HOW THIS BOOK IS ORGANIZED

The 15 priority issues identified above may be grouped into three clusters representing the broad contexts in which today's youth deal with challenges and concerns that many of them share in spite of the vast differences in their cultures, societies and communities. The book is divided into three parts based on these clusters; each starts with an overview of global trends relating to the relevant priority issues, after which one topic is examined in much greater depth. The three clusters are described in some detail below.

Part I: Youth in a Global Economy. This first cluster comprises the issues of globalization, education, employment, and hunger and poverty. Chapter 1 presents an overview of global trends relating to all four issues, and chapters 2 and 3 provide a more in-depth look at young people in poverty.

While poverty reduction is clearly a vitally important development goal, little is known about the dynamics characterizing the poverty situation of young people. In the 2003 *Report*, a first attempt was made to estimate the number of young people living in poverty based on the established thresholds of US$ 1 and US$ 2 per day; in the present publication these figures are updated, and some additional observations are offered. Another (often overlooked) aspect of poverty addressed in this section is the transfer of poverty between generations. In our ageing world, a better understanding of intergenerational dynamics is essential for the development of effective policy interventions.

Part II: Youth in Civil Society. The second part of the publication focuses on concerns relating to the environment, leisure, participation in decision-making, intergenerational relations, and ICT. Chapter 4 provides an overview of global trends with regard to these five issues, and chapters 5 and 6 highlight the impact of ICT on young people's socialization and activism within a changing media landscape.

Growing reliance on new forms of information and communication technology is a defining feature of the lives of many of today's youth. ICT developments have provided young people with an ever-expanding array of media possibilities for obtaining information, pursuing pleasure, and strengthening autonomy. The Internet has been a particularly important component of the ICT revolution for young people. As these media and their "global" content have become more widely accessible, a somewhat homogeneous global youth culture has emerged that binds the world's young people together in important new ways. These technological advances have contributed to a redefinition of some of the most fundamental aspects of society. Most notably, the openness and availability of new technologies have expanded the possibilities for young people to share their views and experiences and contribute to their own cultural development, leading to an increasingly bidirectional flow of socialization between the younger and older generations.

Part III: Youth at Risk. This final cluster encompasses the issues of health, HIV/AIDS, drug abuse, juvenile delinquency, the situation of girls and young women, and youth in armed conflict. A brief summary of recent findings concerning these areas of priority is provided in chapter 7. It should be emphasized, with regard to the issues of health and gender, that young people's basic rights include access to medical care, to information on sexual and reproductive health, and to gender equality, and it is on this basis that policies and programmes should be developed. Chapter 8 focuses on the rise in violent conflict around the world and examines its dramatic impact on young people through a gender lens.

The end of the cold war has not brought about a reduction in armed conflict; on the contrary, many new conflicts have emerged in recent decades, most notably in sub-Saharan Africa but also in other parts of the world. Disproportionate numbers of young people are involved in these conflicts both as perpetrators and as victims. The situation of child soldiers has, deservedly, been widely documented, and a number of international legal instruments incorporating various preventive and protective measures have been adopted to address this issue; unfortunately, these instruments do not protect young people over the age of 18. The rise in armed conflict, terrorism and the threat of terrorism has focused world attention on young males and their potential for violence. As a consequence, the experiences and capacities of young males and females who do not participate in, but are affected by, armed conflicts are marginalized, as are the concerns of female youth who are actively involved in armed violence.

While it may not be immediately apparent, there are some important connections between the issues highlighted in this edition of the *World Youth Report*. First, it may be argued that all three issues — youth in poverty, the emergence of a global media-driven youth culture, and youth in armed conflict — received insufficient attention in the past but have become more central to the wider development interests of the international community. Second, poverty, global youth cultures, and armed conflict are all either directly or indirectly related to globalization. Third, both established and emerging media have made young people increasingly aware of the problems of their peers who are trapped in poverty or in conflict-or both. Fourth, poverty, global youth cultures and armed conflict have a dramatic impact on traditional socialization patterns, affecting families, communities, schools, and other institutions that provide young people with the support they need during their transition to adulthood. Too many young people continue to see promising educational careers cut short by conflict and poverty.

Finally, all three issues reflect aspects of the global divide between young people: there are those who are trapped in poverty and those who are not; there are young people who benefit from new technologies in their lives and careers and young people who lack access to them; and there are youth who can pursue their dreams in a stable environment of peace and security, and those unfortunate enough to become trapped in armed conflict. These disparities and inequalities between the young people of the world need to be eliminated; it is hoped that this book will contribute to a better understanding of where to start. ●

YOUTH

in a

GLOBAL
ECONOMY

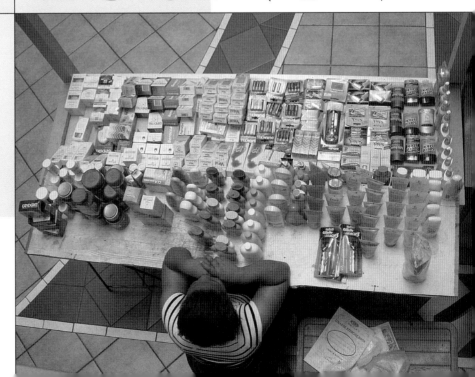

GLOBAL
TRENDS

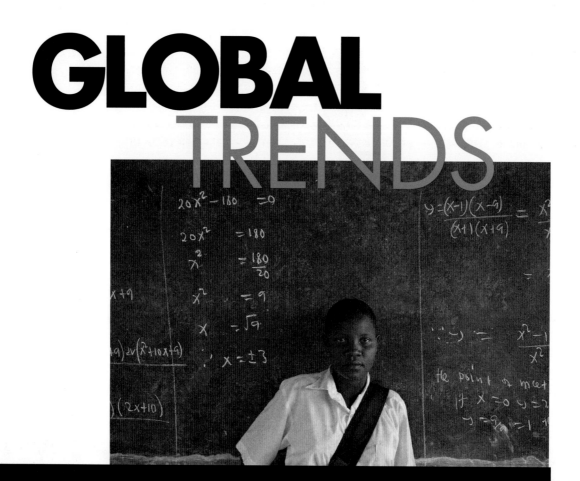

Chapter 1

Global market forces are playing an increasingly impor-
*tant role in determining the prospects for poverty reduction, quality
education, and decent work for all young people. Access to quality
education, decent employment and a life without poverty is to a large
extent determined by the ability of communities and countries to
participate in the global economy. For this reason, youth development
cannot be considered separately from the wider development picture.*

Globalization has an economic, social and cultural impact on all sectors of society. Poverty
cannot be analysed without taking into account the effects of the growing interconnectedness
and interaction within and between countries and regions. Some have clearly benefited
from the increased interdependence; in East Asia, for example, significant economic
growth lifted over 200 million people out of poverty in a single decade. However, there are
many who remain outside the realm of global economic activity and are being left behind;
within and between countries, the income gap is widening (World Commission on the
Social Dimension of Globalization, 2004). About 2 billion people are not benefiting from
globalization, especially in parts of sub-Saharan Africa, Western Asia, and the former Soviet
Union (World Bank, 2004). A number of countries in these regions have experienced declining economic growth, the loss of employment, and persistently low incomes, poor education, and inadequate health provision (United Nations, 2004b; Collier and Dollar, 2001).

Among the 15 areas of policy priority identified in the World Programme of Action
for Youth and General Assembly resolution 58/133 of 2003, globalization, education,
employment, and poverty and hunger relate to the globalized economy and are therefore
addressed in part I of this publication. The characteristics of young people in hunger and
poverty are explored in greater detail in chapters 2 and 3; the second chapter presents an
in-depth analysis of the dimensions and policy implications of youth in extreme poverty,
while the third chapter covers chronic and life-course poverty and the intergenerational
transmission of poverty.

GLOBALIZATION

Young people have an ambiguous economic and cultural relationship with the globalizing
world. They are relatively adaptable and therefore perhaps best able to make use of the
new opportunities presented; they are the best-educated generation, particularly in areas
relating to new information and communication technology (ICT); they benefit from
economic growth; many travel around the globe for work, studies, exchange projects and
vacations; and the telephone and Internet enable them to stay in touch with friends and
relatives all over the world (Boswell and Crisp, 2004). There are still many young people,
however, especially in developing countries, who lack the economic power to benefit from
the opportunities globalization offers. They have been left out of the modernization process
and remain on the other side of the digital divide, but are simultaneously finding their
cultural identity and local traditions threatened.

The challenge for policymakers is to support youth with programmes and policies
that provide them with ICT access and empower them to take advantage of the opportunities and benefits offered by globalization, but that also protect them from its negative

consequences. Some of the issues relevant to the lives of young people in this context, including the distribution of employment opportunities, migration, global consumerism, and participation in anti-globalization movements, are examined in greater detail below.

Globalization has brought about substantial changes in the job market to which young people, as newcomers, may be particularly vulnerable. New technologies have replaced manual labour in a number of industries, mainly affecting low-skill jobs in the manufacturing and service sectors. Even in China, which has experienced remarkable economic growth, unemployment is rising owing to the progressive shift from agriculture to less employment-intensive manufacturing and service industries, the reform of State-owned enterprises, and the reorganization of the public sector (World Commission on the Social Dimension of Globalization, 2004; International Labour Organization, 2004b). Trade liberalization has forced companies to become more flexible and competitive. Many have grown increasingly dependent on low-cost, flexible labour, often employed on an irregular basis. Jobs ranging from semi-skilled work in call centres to sophisticated programming assignments are increasingly being transferred to low-wage countries; this represents perhaps the best-known example of the global shift in employment opportunities for young people (Chowdhury, 2002).

Young people have always constituted a significant proportion of migrant workers. Foreign investment often creates job opportunities in and around cities, inducing rural workers to move to urban areas. In 2003, 48 per cent of the global population lived in urban areas, and this figure is projected to rise to more than 50 per cent by 2007 (United Nations, 2004a). In 2002, there were 175 million international migrants. Most migration data are not disaggregated by age (International Labour Organization, 2004b); however, relevant statistics suggest that an estimated 26 million migrants, or around 15 per cent of the total, are youth.[1] Data on the inflows and outflows of young labour migrants would represent a useful contribution to analyses of the global youth employment situation.

Around the world, many young people nurse hopes of seeking their fortunes in richer countries, often motivated by inaccurate information and unrealistically high expectations. Every day, thousands of young people either willingly or unwillingly join the ranks of illegal migrants. A parallel industry of illicit travel agents, job brokers and middlemen has evolved to "assist" these migrants, many of whom are victims of human trafficking (International Organization for Migration, 1997). The past two decades have seen a dramatic increase in the trafficking of girls and young women, who are often lured into prostitution. Young women and girls who are impoverished and uneducated and who may be members of indigenous, ethnic minority, rural or refugee groups are most vulnerable to this form of exploitation (James and Atler, 2003).

In order to discourage youth migration with its attendant risks and disadvantages, Governments need to create viable employment alternatives for young people in their home countries. At a more fundamental level, action must be taken to address root causes such as poverty and thereby contribute to narrowing the inequalities between rich and poor nations (International Organization for Migration, 1997). Efforts are also required to ensure that young people are provided with sufficient education, training and skill development to gain the knowledge and confidence they need to become successful participants in their national labour markets.

Global consumerism is another aspect of globalization that directly affects youth and has a number of implications for youth cultures. Television programmes, music videos and movies produced in Europe and North America comprise an increasingly dominant share of entertainment media content around the world. This is not necessarily leading to the evolution of a single or unified global youth culture, as young people tend to adopt and interpret global products on the basis of their own local cultures and experiences, thereby creating new hybrid cultural forms whose meanings vary according to local and national circumstances. However, globalization has raised hopes and expectations of increased material well-being. It is feared that constant exposure to images of Western lifestyles and role models may lead to tensions that are both culturally and socially divisive (World Commission on the Social Dimension of Globalization, 2004). Part II of this publication provides a more in-depth look at the emerging global media-driven youth culture and what it means for today's young people.

Young people around the world are expressing their concerns about the negative consequences of globalization, including environmental degradation and the unequal distribution of income and wealth. The anti-globalization movement has expanded world-wide and comprises a heterogeneous collection of non-governmental organizations (NGOs), student groups, political organizations and civil rights activists. Many young people are not against globalization per se, but are simply appealing for a more equitable distri-bution of the opportunities and benefits deriving from globalization (United Nations, 2005). The movement has embraced a broad and eclectic range of issues, including global justice, fair trade, debt relief, and sustainable development.

EDUCATION

Primary school completion rates have continued to climb since 1995. Gross secondary enrolment has risen from 56 to 78 per cent over the past decade (United Nations Educational, Scientific and Cultural Organization, 2004). Global tertiary enrolment increased from 69 million in 1990 to 88 million in 1997, with the most substantial growth achieved in developing countries (United Nations Educational, Scientific and Cultural Organization, 2003a).[2] Some countries even doubled their net enrolment rates during the 1990s. As mentioned previously, today's young people comprise the most highly educated generation in human history.

Unfortunately, some countries have not been as successful as others in providing education for their young people. A few countries experienced declining enrolment during the 1990s and have registered only moderate increases in the past five years. Some of the transition economies have suffered a regression in primary education, suggesting that achieving basic education for all is tied to socio-economic circumstances. In spite of the overall progress achieved, 113 million primary-school-age children around the world were not in school in 2000 (United Nations Educational, Scientific and Cultural Organization/ Institute for Statistics, 2000). These children will become the next generation of illiterate youth, taking the place of the estimated 130 million illiterate youth of today as they enter adulthood and the job market — already at a serious disadvantage.

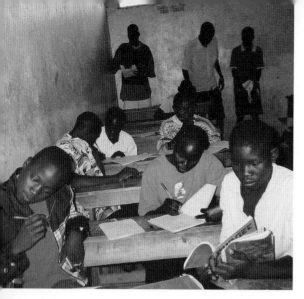

Poverty remains a major barrier to schooling, and gender discrimination is a factor as well. When poor parents need to make a choice about which of their children should receive an education, girls tend to be excluded first. The literacy gap between young men and young women appears to be widening in Africa and Asia; the greatest gender inequalities are found in North Africa and Western Asia, where educationally deprived girls outnumber the corresponding groups of boys by almost three to one.[3] Countries in East Asia and Pacific have come close to achieving gender parity in access to education, while in Latin America and the Caribbean there appears to be a slight bias against boys. In rural areas, young people have less access to education, the quality of education is poorer, and adult illiteracy rates are higher.

The most important challenge, apart from achieving education for all, is ensuring the provision of a quality education. Many countries have abolished school fees, and while such a move stimulates school enrolment, it can have negative implications for the quality of education. Experience in various sub-Saharan African countries has shown that without additional funding for qualified teachers and material resources, schools are unable to accommodate the larger numbers of students seeking an education. Teachers and trainers in many parts of the world lack sufficient training, resources, support, materials, and conducive conditions of service, which adversely affects young people's learning experience. In pursuing the goal of a quality education for all, the importance of teachers and trainers must be recognized. Attention should be given to their education, professional development, wages, working conditions, and career paths in order to make teaching a more attractive option.

New approaches are needed to respond to the evolving educational needs of youth, especially in the light of the ongoing technological revolution and the global inequalities it has engendered. Educational curricula are not always in line with the demands of the labour market, and young people may find themselves inadequately prepared for the world of work. It has been estimated that in developed countries, roughly 10 to 20 per cent of the general population's learning needs are not adequately met by the current formal learning systems (United Nations Educational, Scientific and Cultural Organization, 2003b). Developing countries face major challenges in introducing new ICT in the education system. Urgent attention is needed to prevent the digital divide between developed and developing countries from widening in the next generation.

Education has long been regarded as one of the primary components of poverty reduction efforts and overall social development. The World Declaration on Education for All, adopted in Jomtien, Thailand, in 1990, affirmed the international commitment to universalizing primary education and massively reducing illiteracy before the end of the decade. In the World Programme of Action for Youth to the Year 2000 and Beyond, education is listed first among the 10 priority areas for youth development. The Dakar Framework for Action, adopted at the World Education Forum in 2000, identified six major goals for education, two of which became Millennium Development Goals (MDGs) later that year. The two Goals incorporate the following targets: (a) ensure that by 2015, all children will be able to complete a full course of primary schooling; and (b) eliminate gender disparities in primary and secondary education, preferably by 2005, and at all levels of education by no later than 2015.

In a number of major international projects and activities, specific strategies are being employed to achieve the MDGs. The Millennium Project, launched by the Secretary-General of the United Nations, has task forces focusing on education. In 2002, the World Bank launched the Fast Track Initiative to provide immediate and incremental technical and financial support to countries that have appropriate educational policies but are not on track to achieve universal primary education by 2015. Nine flagship inter-agency programmes have been put in place by UNESCO. Although there have been some positive developments in financing basic education, both bilateral and multilateral aid to education decreased between 1998/99 and 2000/01 (United Nations Educational, Scientific and Cultural Organization, 2003b). The current level of international assistance appears to be insufficient to achieve universal primary education by 2015.

Most countries guarantee the right to education in their constitutions. Ultimately, however, real progress will depend on the extent to which educational rights and commitments translate into enforceable legislation and well-conceived policies, plans and programmes. The Dakar Framework for Action requests States to develop or strengthen national action plans for education and to ensure that they are integrated into wider poverty reduction and development frameworks (World Education Forum, 2000). Many Governments are setting specific national education goals, including gender-related targets. Over the past decade, NGOs have increasingly campaigned for education and contributed to its delivery, benefiting millions of young people.

Various countries have integrated programmes in their educational curricula that address racism and violence, promote multicultural values and tolerance, and allow youth to be educated in their native languages.

In the past decade there has been a growing emphasis on "life competencies" within the education system. The rising popularity of alternative approaches and modalities such as non-formal learning, lifelong learning, distance education, e-learning, peer education and on-the-job training shows that the concept of education is increasingly expanding beyond the traditional classroom. It is important that efforts be made to reach youth and young adults who have dropped out of the formal education system before acquiring basic literacy and numeracy skills and provide them with education or training that will enhance their employability. Governments are encouraged to establish systems to ensure the recognition, validation and accreditation of non-formal and informal learning for young people. Such a move would acknowledge the value of knowledge and experience gained outside of the traditional learning environment, and demonstrate the importance of integrating formal and non-formal learning in overall educational provision.

International efforts to promote education have mainly targeted girls and young women. Continuing efforts should be made to sustain the positive trend towards gender parity and equality in education and subsequently in employment. There is evidence that educated girls and young women are better able to make decisions that enhance their well-being and improve the lives of any children they may have. Public policy measures that have proved successful and should be promoted include creating an enabling environment for advancing female education through legislative and policy reforms; redistributing resources to meet girls' specific educational needs; reforming curricula; providing incentives to families that make sending all children to school a worthwhile proposition; increasing the number of educational facilities in underserved areas; improving teacher training; confronting violence; working with parents; instituting school feeding programmes; increasing the presence of female teachers; separating sanitation facilities and providing privacy for girls; furnishing school-based health education; and raising the minimum legal age of marriage. Such interventions require a strong public commitment from the State, though the support of non-State actors is essential as well.

EMPLOYMENT

Labour force participation rates for young people decreased by almost four percentage points between 1993 and 2003, largely as a result of the increased numbers of young people attending school, the tendency of students to remain in the education system for a longer period, high overall unemployment rates, and the fact that some young people gave up any hope of finding work and dropped out of the labour market. Figures published by the International Labour Organization (ILO) indicate that global youth unemployment increased from 11.7 per cent in 1993 to an all-time high of 14.4 per cent (88 million) in 2003.[4] At the regional level, youth unemployment was highest in Western Asia and North Africa (25.6 per cent) and sub-Saharan Africa (21 per cent), and lowest in East Asia (7 per cent) and the industrialized economies (13.4 per cent). There is a general trend towards the convergence of male and female labour force participation rates, though unemployment rates are still higher for women than for men in all developing regions except East Asia and sub-Saharan Africa. Thanks to the concerted efforts of Governments, civil society and the international community, child labour appears to be on the decline throughout the world.

The increase in the numbers of youth in secondary and tertiary education is a positive development; however, labour markets in many countries are presently unable to accommodate the expanding pools of skilled young graduates. In a number of settings this is partially attributable to the failure to coordinate education provision with labour market needs, but it is perhaps more fundamentally linked to the fact that large numbers of youth are now coming of age and are trying to find work. In the absence of opportunities in the formal labour market, many young people resort to "forced entrepreneurship" and self-employment in the informal economy, often working for low pay under hazardous conditions, with few prospects for the future. Together, these factors can cause disillusionment and alienation among younger workers. As mentioned previously, young people also constitute a significant proportion of the 175 million global migrants, which contributes to the brain drain in their home countries (United Nations, 2003).

There has been increasing concern among policymakers that the frustrations accompanying long-term unemployment among groups of urban young men may feed political and ideological unrest and provoke violence (Commission for Africa, 2005). Many countries have experienced "youth bulges", which occur when young people comprise at least 40 per cent of the population, and it has been argued that in such a context, the large

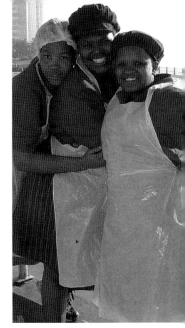

numbers of unemployed and idle youth may challenge the authority of the Government and endanger its stability (inter alia; Urdal, 2004; Cincotta, Engelman and Anastasion, 2003). The contention is that these disaffected individuals are more likely to participate in national and international conflicts. However, the fact is that only a very small number of people engage in such activities, and many are not members of the younger generation.

Over the past decade, the international community has strengthened its commitment to addressing youth employment. In 1995, Governments called for special attention to youth unemployment in the Copenhagen Declaration on Social Development and Programme of Action of the World Summit for Social Development (United Nations, 1995). Six years later, youth organizations adopted the Dakar Youth Empowerment Strategy at the fourth session of the World Youth Forum of the United Nations System (Dakar Youth Empowerment Strategy, 2001). [5] The United Nations Millennium Declaration, adopted by the General Assembly in 2000, reflects the commitment of heads of State and Government to develop and implement strategies that give young people everywhere real opportunities to find decent and productive work. This objective was subsequently integrated into the MDGs (United Nations, 2000); the eighth Goal, which relates to developing a global partnership for development, explicitly refers to creating employment opportunities for young people. The Youth Employment Network (YEN), comprising the United Nations, ILO and World Bank as core partners, was established following the Millennium Summit to initiate action on the ground, with the result that the youth employment issue has gained momentum at the national level. Recommendations based on four global policy priorities — employability, entrepreneurship, equal opportunities for young women and men, and employment creation—were issued in 2001 by the High-Level Panel on Youth Employment, a team of experts appointed by the Secretary-General. The YEN is now supporting the efforts of 13 lead countries committed to the development and execution of strategies for youth employment, as well as those of a number of other countries currently at various stages in the planning or implementation of national action plans in this context.[6]

At the national level, several of the Poverty Reduction Strategy Papers[7] recently completed by developing countries have outlined youth employment strategies focusing on youth entrepreneurship training, microcredit schemes, the development of vocational training and career guidance services, youth leadership training, youth-targeted labour-intensive programmes, and the acquisition of ICT skills. In addition, several national human development reports have been devoted entirely to youth, and others have included sections dedicated to national youth employment initiatives and policies.

Although many Governments encourage entrepreneurship and self-employment among youth at the conceptual level, relatively few microfinancing initiatives specifically targeted at young people have emerged on the ground. Microfinancing schemes are usually implemented by NGOs or private banks. A number of NGOs have set up programmes to enhance life skills, provide job training, and develop entrepreneurial skills among youth. Many initiatives that have been undertaken are too small in terms of both scale and resources to address the full scope of the youth unemployment problem. There is a need, at both the national and international levels, to scale up the successful aspects of these initiatives if they are to have a real impact on poverty reduction. Therefore, it is essential that financial commitments to youth employment initiatives be substantially increased.

HUNGER AND POVERTY

It is generally agreed that poverty is multidimensional and should be measured not only by income, but also by access to public goods such as education, health care, a safe water supply, and adequate roads (Gordon and others, 2003; also see World Bank, 2004). This perspective should be applied in the formulation of youth development strategies, with steps taken to move beyond the limited focus on monetary indicators towards the adoption of a more comprehensive approach to addressing the full range of problems faced by poor young people. An integrated approach should reflect consideration of all the priority areas for youth development (identified in the World Programme of Action for Youth and General Assembly resolution 58/133 of 2003) that may be relevant to young people in their local and national contexts. Further, the youth component should form part of a broader national pro-poor growth strategy that includes infrastructure development and agricultural policy changes aimed at helping those in poverty (Hoddinott and Quisumbing, 2003).

Not much is known about the numbers of poor young people around the world and the ways they experience poverty. There are no specific references to youth in the targets or indicators of the MDG relating to hunger and poverty, and very little age-disaggregated poverty data are available. Few researchers have looked into the poverty characteristics of young people and their movement in and out of poverty. Most youth are relatively healthy, live with and receive support from their families, benefit from an extensive education, and do not yet have children to take care of. However, many young people have suffered deprivation during childhood, are affected by HIV/AIDS, have full responsibility for the care of their siblings, marry and have children before the age of 25, or are unemployed. All youth are in a transition period, moving towards independence and adulthood. During this stage of their lives, they face a multitude of challenges that tend to compound any other difficulties they may be experiencing. The capacity to make a successful transition to adulthood is shaped by the society in which a person lives and by a complex combination of factors such as gender, socio-economic background, family support, ethnicity, and race (Curtain, 2004). Governments need to identify the challenges faced by young people in their countries and to develop policies and programmes that help them make a smooth transition to adulthood.

In the *World Youth Report, 2003*, the observation was made that young people had been neglected in poverty reduction strategies, in part because there was little poverty research focused specifically on young people and a consequent lack of relevant data disaggregated by age. Some approximate figures were derived by the author based on different measures of poverty; it was estimated that 110.1 million young people were undernourished, 238 million were living on less than US$ 1 a day, and 462 million were living on less than US$ 2 a day (United Nations, 2004b). However, these calculations were based on the assumption that poverty in a country was evenly distributed among all age groups in the population. It was concluded that further quantitative and qualitative research on poverty alleviation among youth was needed to provide a better understanding of the poverty dynamics for this group. In the coming chapters, this argument is reiterated. Because the static definition of poverty provides only a limited picture, emphasis is given to the importance of longitudinal data studies that monitor poverty dynamics over time. This kind of data would provide a sounder basis for anti-poverty policy formulation than would reliance on poverty trend data alone.

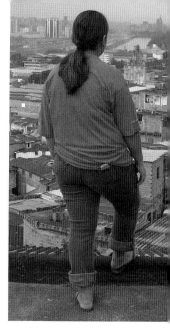

Chapter 2 offers a deeper analysis of the dimensions and policy implications of extreme poverty among youth. It is argued that young people in poverty will not be given the attention they deserve in national poverty reduction strategies until their situation is formally acknowledged, they are consulted, and data are available on the nature and extent of their vulnerabilities. The methods and indicators currently used by international agencies and Governments to measure poverty are examined. It is noted that data on youth in poverty are scarce, there is no global measurement to assess youth development over time, and most countries do not involve young people in the design or implementation of poverty reduction strategies. New estimates of the numbers of young people living in poverty are provided, and suggestions are made regarding the development of pro-poor growth strategies that include young people as a focus group and as partners.

Chapter 3 focuses on the concepts of chronic poverty, life-course poverty and the intergenerational transmission of poverty as they relate to youth poverty. An intergenerational perspective adds a critical dimension in assessing and addressing global poverty. It is argued that the extent to which a young person is economically dependent, independent, or depended upon within the household can change extremely rapidly. This has significant implications for the present and long-term well-being of both young people and their families. Interventions in the areas of education, health and employment can break the poverty cycle; without such interventions, poverty tends to deepen with age and over successive generations. ●

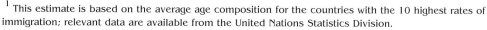

[1] This estimate is based on the average age composition for the countries with the 10 highest rates of immigration; relevant data are available from the United Nations Statistics Division.

[2] The rate of entry into tertiary education increased by 50 per cent in developing countries between 1990 and 1997 (rising from 29 million to 43.4 million), while the increase in developed countries was much slower (rising by only 13 per cent, from 39.5 million to 44.8 million) during this period; 1997 is the last year for which worldwide data are available and comparable with earlier statistics. Since 1997, different categories for the International Standard Classification of Education have been used, affecting the comparability of statistics for secondary and tertiary education (United Nations Educational, Scientific and Cultural Organization, 2003a, p. 68).

[3] The designation "severely educationally deprived" refers to children between the ages of 7 and 18 who have not had any primary or secondary education (those who have never attended school) (see Gordon and others, 2003).

[4] Unemployment rates take into account only those who are looking for work; they do not include those who are discouraged and have stopped looking or have not looked for work, or those who have voluntarily remained in education and training (International Labour Organization, 2004b, p. 12).

[5] Also see the letter of the Government of Senegal to the United Nations General Assembly conveying the results of the Fourth World Youth Forum, cited in A/C.3/56/2.

[6] The 13 countries include Azerbaijan, Brazil, Egypt, Indonesia, the Islamic Republic of Iran, Mali, Namibia, Nigeria, Rwanda, Senegal, Sri Lanka, the Syrian Arab Republic and the United Kingdom.

[7] "Poverty Reduction Strategy Papers (PRSPs) describe a country's macroeconomic, structural and social policies and programmes to promote growth and reduce poverty, as well as associated external financing needs. PRSPs are prepared by Governments through a participatory process involving civil society and development partners, including the World Bank and the International Monetary Fund (IMF)."

Bibliography

Boswell, C., and J. Crisp (2004). *Poverty, International Migration and Asylum.* Helsinki: United Nations University/World Institute for Development Economics Research.

Chowdhury, N. (2002). *The Information Revolution and Globalization: Seizing New Opportunities for Youth Employment.* New York: The Century Foundation, Inc.

Cincotta, R., R. Engelman and D. Anastasion (2003). *The Security Demographic: Population and Civil Conflict After the Cold War.* Washington, D.C.: Population Action International.

Collier, P., and D. Dollar (2001). *Globalization, Growth and Poverty: Building an Inclusive World Economy.* Washington, D.C., and New York: World Bank and Oxford University Press.

Commission for Africa (2005). *Our Common Interest: Report of the Commission for Africa.* March.

Curtain, R. (2004). The case for investing in young people as part of a national poverty reduction strategy. Paper commissioned by the United Nations Population Fund for the Technical Meeting on Promoting Sexual and Reproductive Health and Reproductive Rights: Reducing Poverty and Achieving the MDGs, Stockholm, 5-6 October.

Dakar Youth Empowerment Strategy (2001). Adopted during the Fourth World Youth Forum of the United Nations System, Dakar, 5-10 August.

Gordon, D., and others (2003). *Child Poverty in the Developing World.* Bristol, United Kingdom: The Policy Press.

Hoddinott, J., and A. Quisumbing (2003). Investing in children and youth for poverty reduction. Washington, D.C.: International Food Policy Research Institute. 24 June.

International Labour Organization (2004a). *Global Employment Trends.* Geneva.

_____ (2004b). *Global Employment Trends for Youth.* Geneva.

International Organization for Migration (1997). *Trafficking in Migrants: Quarterly Bulletin*, No. 13 (March).

James, C., and S. Atler (2003). Trafficking of young women. In *Highly Affected, Rarely Considered: The International Youth Parliament Commission's Report on the Impacts of Globalisation on Young People.* Sydney: Oxfam International Youth Parliament.

United Nations (1995). Report of the World Summit for Social Development, Copenhagen, 6-12 March 1995. A/CONF.166/9. 19 April 1995.

_____ (1995). World Programme of Action for Youth to the Year 2000 and Beyond. A/RES/50/81. 14 December.

_____ (2000). United Nations Millennium Declaration. General Assembly resolution 55/2 of 8 September. A/RES/55/2. 18 September.

_____ (2003). *Trends in Total Migrant Stock: The 2003 Revision* (available from http://www.un.org/esa/population/publications/migstock/2003TrendsMigstock.pdf.)

_____ (2004a). *World Urbanization Prospects: The 2003 Revision.* Sales No. E.04.XIII.6.

_____ (2004b). *World Youth Report, 2003: The Global Situation of Young People.* Sales No. E.03.IV.7, pp. 78-82 and 292-293.

_____ (2005). Report and recommendations of the Meeting. Outcome document from the Consultative Meeting on the 10-Year Review of the World Programme of Action for Youth, Coimbra, Portugal, 31 January to 3 February.

United Nations Educational, Scientific and Cultural Organization (1990). World Declaration on Education for All and Framework for Action to Meet Basic Learning Needs. Adopted by the World Conference on Education for All. Meeting basic Learning Needs. Jomtien, Thailand, 5-9 March. New York

_____ (2003a). *Education for All Global Monitoring Report, 2003/04 — Gender and Education for All: The Leap to Equality.* Paris.

_____ (2003b). Education for All Global Monitoring Report, 2003/04 — Gender and Education for All: The Leap to Equality, summary report. Paris.

_____ (2004). Quality education for all young people: challenges, trends and priorities. Paris, p. 6. Citing the *Education for All Global Monitoring Report, 2003/04 — Gender and Education for All: The Leap to Equality.*

_____, Institute for Statistics (2000). *Education for All Year 2000 Assessment: Statistical Document.* Report for the International Consultative Forum on Education for All, World Education Forum, Dakar, 26-28 April. Paris. Cited in United Nations, *World Youth Report 2003: The Global Situation of Young People.* Sales No. E.03.IV.7.

Urdal, H. (2004). The devil in the demographics: the effect of youth bulges on domestic armed conflict, 1950-2000. Social Development Papers, Conflict Prevention & Reconstruction, Paper No. 14. Washington, D.C.: World Bank. July.

World Bank (2004). Shanghai agenda on poverty reduction. Working Conference on Scaling Up Poverty Reduction: A Global Learning Process, Shanghai, China, 25-27 May (available from www.world-bank.org/wbi/reducingpoverty/docs/confDocs/ShanghaiAgenda-FinalVersion.pdf).

World Commission on the Social Dimension of Globalization (2004). *A Fair Globalization: Creating Opportunities for All.* Geneva: International Labour Organization.

World Education Forum (2000). The Dakar Framework for Action—*Education for All: Meeting Our Collective Commitments.* Paris: United Nations Educational, Scientific and Cultural Organization.

YOUNG PEOPLE IN POVERTY:

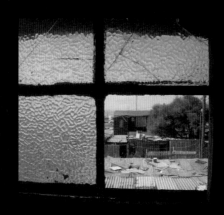

dimensions

and

policy implications

Chapter 2

Many young people in the world experience extreme poverty, though there is little published evidence to confirm this fact. The present chapter outlines the best ways, from the perspective of national public policy, to identify young people in poverty. It provides estimates of youth living on less than US$ 1 and US$ 2 a day in 2002. Because of the limitations associated with income-based measures of absolute poverty, estimates of the numbers of young people in hunger, based on 1999-2001 data, are also presented.

Poverty in developing countries affects most residents in that it diminishes life chances. It is impossible to develop comprehensive national poverty reduction strategies without reliable information on the prevalence of poverty among groups such as young women or rural youth that have been excluded from the benefits of economic growth in the past. It is important to identify young people as a distinct group experiencing extreme poverty to ensure that issues of specific relevance to them are addressed in poverty reduction strategies. Access to reliable data also makes it much easier for young people to participate in formulating or refining national poverty reduction strategies.

Some politicians and analysts argue that a rising tide will float all boats, meaning that economic growth alone is sufficient to reduce poverty. However, this view is increasingly being challenged, as there is evidence that the relationship between economic growth and poverty reduction is neither simple nor direct. It is only when Governments and other stakeholders have made a concerted effort to direct resources to those identified as poorer than their peers that both economic growth and poverty reduction have been achieved (Pernia, 2003).

DEFINITION OF TERMS
Young People

Defining youth as those between the ages of 15 and 24 is a widely accepted statistical convention, and it is this group that constitutes the focus of the present chapter. It is much harder to specify a set age group when a sociological definition of young people is employed. The period of transition from childhood to adulthood varies greatly between societies and even within the same society. This critical stage in the life cycle may begin as early as age 10 (for street children, for example) and may in some cases continue into the mid- to late 30s. The Youth Policy Act in India, for instance, defines the group it addresses as ranging in age from 15 to 35 (Brown and Larson, 2002). This relatively wide age span suggests that the process of achieving an independent, sustaining livelihood can take a relatively long time, particularly in poor societies.

Measuring poverty

It is not possible to determine the extent of poverty among young people until a consensus is reached on how poverty should be measured. Such an exercise is fraught with difficulties. The first challenge is defining the concept of poverty itself. Is it merely a lack of income, or does it also reflect deficiencies in other dimensions of human survival and well-being such as access to adequate sanitation, health care and educational opportunities? If poverty is defined more broadly, what measures are appropriate to ensure access to needed services? In relation to the poverty measures used, should the reference point be some absolute level, or is poverty a relative concept that needs to be defined based on the standard of living of the society in which the poor live?

The Millennium Development Goals (MDGs) and targets resolve much of the ambivalence surrounding the measurement of poverty. The MDGs acknowledge the multi-dimensional nature of poverty and establish benchmarks not only for increasing income levels but also for improving access to food, basic education and literacy, educational opportunities for girls, quality health care, and adequate sanitation in the form of good drinking water. The Millennium Declaration and the MDGs reflect the international consensus on the importance of poverty eradication as a major development objective.

It is now widely accepted that income is not the only measure of poverty (Hulme and Shepherd, 2003). The Poverty Reduction Strategy Paper (PRSP) prepared by the Government of Mozambique provides an illustrative example of the broader concept, noting that poverty encompasses not only income deficiency but also the lack of human capacities, manifested in "illiteracy, malnutrition, low life expectancy, poor maternal health, (and the) prevalence of preventable diseases", and is also reflected in indirect measures indicating a lack of access to the "goods, services and infrastructures necessary to achieve basic human capacities, (including) sanitation, clean drinking water, education, communications, (and) energy" (Mozambique, 2001, p. 11).

This broader view of poverty has evolved largely owing to the work of Nobel Laureate Amartya Sen, who contends that poverty is best understood as various forms of "unfreedom" that prevent people from realizing and expanding their capabilities. From this perspective, civil and political liberties and economic and social rights are viewed as primary goals of development and the principal means of progress (International Labour Organization, 2003).

The need for a dynamic view of poverty

It is implied, within this broader context, that poverty is both a static and a dynamic phenomenon. In other words, it is a state people experience that can change according to circumstances. The dynamic view of poverty is often particularly relevant to young people, given the obstacles most of them face in endeavouring to achieve independent adult status. The dynamic view of poverty starts from the premise that the "determining condition for poor people is uncertainty" (Wood, 2003). Young people's capacities to cope with uncertainties are shaped by a range of supports, including the legal rights, entitlements and support systems provided by Governments and employers. They are also influenced by personal attributes and achievements such as educational attainment and physical health (Wood, 2003). The best policy responses in such circumstances involve the provision of various forms of social protection to help the poor cope with the unexpected.

Young people and the Millennium Development Goals

Most of the MDGs relate to challenges young people are facing. Around 51 per cent of the combined population of developing and least developed countries are below the age of 25, and 20 per cent are 15 to 24 years of age (United Nations, 2005b). It is clear, given such age demographics, that if the specific needs of young people are not identified and addressed, the MDGs will not be met.

Young people per se do not appear to have a prominent place in the MDGs. However, on closer scrutiny, five of the Goals may be identified as referring directly to youth because they relate to issues primarily associated with young people, including educational attainment, gender balance in education, improved maternal health, combating HIV/AIDS and other diseases such as malaria and tuberculosis, and decent employment opportunities for youth (*see table 2.1*).

Greater investment in improving adolescent health and education will not only reduce poverty, but will also bring countries closer to achieving the targets for two other MDGs. Overall improvements in adolescent health will reduce the incidence of high-risk pregnancies among undernourished teenagers and thereby contribute significantly to reducing child mortality, the objective of Goal 4. Higher educational levels and improved nutrition among young mothers will help reduce the prevalence of underweight children below five years of age (one of the indicators for Goal 1), which will contribute substantially to the eradication of hunger, as called for in Goal 1.

Table 2.1
Millennium Development Goals, targets and indicators
relating to young people

Goal	Target	Indicator
1. Eradicate extreme poverty and hunger	1. Halve, between 1990 and 2015, the proportion of people whose income is less than US$ 1 a day 2. Halve, between 1990 and 2015, the proportion of people who suffer from hunger	1. Proportion of the population living on less than US$ 1 a day (1993 purchasing power parity) 4. Prevalence of underweight children under five years of age
2. Achieve universal primary education	3. Ensure that, by 2015, children everywhere, boys and girls alike, will be able to complete a full course of primary schooling	8. Literacy rate of 15- to 24-year olds
3. Promote gender equality and empower women	4. Eliminate gender disparity in primary and secondary education, preferably by 2005, and in all levels of education no later than 2015	9. Ratio of girls to boys in primary, secondary and tertiary education 10. Ratio of literate women to men 15-24 years old
5. Improve maternal health	6. Reduce by three quarters, between 1990 and 2015, the maternal mortality ratio	16. Maternal mortality ratio
6. Combat HIV/AIDS, malaria and other diseases	7. Have halted by 2015 and begun to reverse the spread of HIV/AIDS	18. HIV prevalence among pregnant women aged 15-24 years
8. Develop a global partnership for development	16. In cooperation with developing countries, develop and implement strategies for decent and productive work for youth	45. Unemployment rate of young people aged 15-24 years, each sex and total

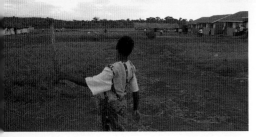

The prominence of young people in the MDGs is further confirmed by the fact that they constitute the explicit or implicit focus of seven targets and eight indicators (see table 2.1). Four of the performance indicators specifically refer to individuals between the ages of 15 and 24, and two others refer to circumstances that apply to many young people, namely secondary and tertiary education and motherhood.

The poverty measure used for Goal 1 is per capita income, but the relevant indicator does not include any reference to males and females separately. However, four performance indicators refer specifically to girls and young women. Goals 5 and 6 relate to sexual and reproductive health and implicitly target young people, as members of this age group are likely to benefit most from actions undertaken to achieve these Goals. In reference to Goal 5, young women under the age of 25 account for many of those who will benefit from increased investments in improving maternal health. In the least developed countries, for example, females under 20 years of age account for 17 per cent of all births (United Nations Population Fund, 2004). Young people are also potentially the main beneficiaries of actions taken to achieve Goal 6 (combating HIV/AIDS, malaria and other diseases) and one of its targets in particular (halting and beginning to reverse the spread of HIV/AIDS by 2015), as nearly half of all new HIV infections worldwide occur among individuals between the ages of 15 and 24 (Joint United Nations Programme on HIV/AIDS, 2004).

POVERTY AND PUBLIC POLICY

In a conscious effort to move away from narrow income measures of poverty and progress, the United Nations Development Programme has established a framework that includes country-level data on a wide range of social indicators such as life expectancy at birth, under-five mortality, literacy rates, access to clean water, and measures of equity or parity including male-female gaps in schooling and political participation (United Nations Development Programme, various years). These indicators are then converted into summary measures such as the human development index and the human poverty index for developing countries. The aim is to give policymakers comprehensive measures with which to assess their country's progress in terms of overall human well-being and to move away from exclusive reliance on per capita income as a measure of development.

Similarly, a youth development index may be used to assess a country's progress in addressing the social and economic challenges faced by young people. The UNESCO Office in Brazil has created such an index using various education, health and income indicators. The education indicators either comprise or derive from illiteracy rates, the numbers of youth attending secondary and tertiary institutions, and assessments of the quality of education offered to young people. The health indicators reflect mortality rates (deaths from both internal causes and violence). The remaining indicators focus on the per capita income of youth in the country's different federative units. In the data gathering and analysis, distinguishing factors such as place of residence (rural or urban), gender and race are taken into account (Waiselfisz, 2004). The youth development index served as the basis for the *Youth Development Report, 2003*, the first such publication issued by the UNESCO

Office in Brazil to monitor public policies on youth in the country's 27 states. The Government is currently drafting its first national youth policy and is using the findings in the youth development index in its deliberations. Consideration should be given to using the Brazilian index as a model for a global youth development index that could be adapted to reflect different national priorities for youth.

The need for pro-poor growth strategies to reduce poverty

As mentioned previously, the link between economic growth and poverty alleviation is neither simple nor straightforward. Higher income levels are important for reducing poverty, but income disparities do not by themselves account for the differences in poverty levels between countries. This indicates that the poor often do not benefit from economic growth to the same extent as the rest of the population. The connection between economic growth and poverty reduction is largely determined by key inputs such as the types of institutions and specific policies Governments have in place to ensure that the poor benefit more than the population as a whole. Pro-growth strategies need to be distinguished from pro-*poor* growth strategies, as it is only the latter that will bring about substantial reductions in poverty levels (Pernia, 2003).

Pro-poor growth strategies must incorporate a wide range of policies that facilitate comprehensive development. Policies that promote economic openness, a favourable investment climate, efficient resource acquisition and allocation, and appropriate labour market regulations are essential. Equally important, however, are policies that address institutional discrimination against the poor on the basis of gender, ethnicity, religion, or employment within the informal rather than the formal economy (Pernia, 2003; also see World Bank, 2004). Box 2.1 illustrates how Viet Nam has reduced poverty by applying a combination of economic and pro-poor growth strategies.

Box 2.1

PRO-POOR GROWTH STRATEGIES IN VIET NAM

According to a 2003 report by international donor agencies, the progress made by Viet Nam in reducing poverty has been "simply remarkable".[a] Figures for 2002 indicate that the proportion of the population living in poverty was reduced by half in less than a decade.[b] This achievement illustrates how effective pro-poor growth strategies can be. While some regions and population groups have benefited more than others — poverty seems to be persistent in many rural areas and among minority groups, as noted in chapter 3 — Viet Nam continues to reduce poverty considerably faster than other countries at a similar level of development.

The vast improvement in the poverty situation in Viet Nam is the result of both targeted policies to reduce poverty and strong economic growth. Public policies have ensured that the poor are reached through targeted transfers, and the Government has also increased the non-monetary assets of the poor by facilitating higher levels of educational attainment and improved health status. These policies have been greatly reinforced by high rates of economic growth, second only to those of China and Ireland over the past decade. At the same time, challenges such as the country's determined fight against corruption remain on the agenda. It has been acknowledged that the "abuse of public office for private gain risks making everyday life miserable when it happens at low levels", and when it reaches a point where collective decision-making is affected, it can lead to resource misallocation and waste.[c] Improving governance at all levels reduces constraints on both poverty reduction and economic growth.

There are 16 million young people between the ages of 15 and 24 in Viet Nam,[d] approximately 2 million of which are poor. The recently completed Youth Development Strategy to 2010 identifies unemployment as the single greatest challenge currently facing Vietnamese youth, and efforts to address this problem are at the centre of the national fight against poverty. It is estimated that 5 per cent of young people are out of work, and 26 per cent are underemployed.[e] One policy change in Viet Nam that has benefited young people in particular relates to the starting and running of enterprises. Since the enactment of the Enterprise Law in 2000, almost 60,000 private companies have been created in the country, providing 1.3 million to 1.5 million new jobs. The Viet Nam Association of Young Entrepreneurs claims that young businesspeople set up three quarters of the private enterprises established between 2000 and 2002.[f] However, the new jobs are mostly to be found in the main urban centres, as the rural provinces have not benefited from the new Enterprise Law to the same extent. Other regulatory obstacles give State-owned enterprises an advantage over private firms.[g]

The capacity to scale up policies and programmes is an important prerequisite for achieving poverty reduction. "Absorptive capacity" refers to the human resources, managerial skills, monitoring and evaluation systems, and infrastructure available in a country; low absorptive capacity can impose major constraints on a country's ability to expand a successful programme and operate it on a much larger scale. Viet Nam, with its high rates of literacy and numeracy, long experience with mass organizations, and ability to mobilize people down to the village level, has sufficient absorptive capacity to continue moving forward in developing programmes and strategies for reducing poverty.

---

[a] World Bank, *Viet Nam Development Report, 2004: Poverty* (Hanoi, World Bank, 2003), p. xi.

[b] Ibid. In 2002, 29 per cent of the population lived in poverty, compared with 37 per cent in 1998 and 58 per cent in 1993.

[c] Ibid., p. xii.

[d] All figures presented in this paragraph are taken from Vu Van Toan (Viet Nam Ministry of Labour, War Invalids and Social Affairs), "Policies and measures for young in poverty in Viet Nam", a PowerPoint presentation given at the Workshop on Youth in Poverty in Southeast Asia, organized by the United Nations Department of Economic and Social Affairs and held in Yogyakarta, Indonesia, from 2 to 4 August 2004.

[e] United Nations Country Team in Viet Nam, "United Nations message on International Youth Day: tap the energies of youth" (Hanoi, United Nations Development Programme, 12 August 2003).

[f] Thu Ha, "Self-employed youth to tackle unemployment", Viet Nam Investment Review (11-17 August 2003), p. 19.

[g] Ibid.

As illustrated in the case of Viet Nam, pro-poor policies may be incorporated in national poverty reduction strategies. Such policies may include provisions for increased public spending for basic education, improved health and family planning services, easier access to microcredit, the promotion of small and medium-sized enterprises, or infrastructure investments in rural areas (Pernia, 2003).

The neglect of young people in national poverty reduction strategies

Many poor countries are still not giving the needs of young people sufficient priority, as indicated by a review of 31 PRSPs completed prior to August 2003. Although an increasing number of countries are making some reference to young people in their Papers, the initiatives proposed are often piecemeal and therefore limited in terms of scale, scope, and potential impact.

These country strategy papers and accompanying action plans are produced by Governments in heavily indebted countries as a requirement for debt relief. The aim of the PRSP process is to identify all groups experiencing poverty and to highlight cross-cutting issues that contribute to poverty in a country so that national policies can be developed to address these challenges. While the process is designed to produce tailor-made approaches to development, the PRSPs have been criticized for looking strikingly similar, even among countries that face very different challenges (Vandemoortele, 2004).

Most of the PRSPs have been prepared by African countries, though some have come from Asia (Cambodia, Kyrgyzstan, Sri Lanka, Tajikistan and Viet Nam), Europe (Albania and Moldova), and Latin America (Bolivia, Honduras and Nicaragua). While it appears that few Governments consulted young people in the PRSP drafting process or identified youth as a major group experiencing poverty, 17 of the 31 Papers completed between May 2002 and September 2003 do make some mention of youth in their action plans, mainly in relation to education and employment. However, closer scrutiny reveals that only a few of the action plans link youth-focused strategies to specific targets and budget outlays (Rosen, 2003).

There is little evidence that the youth situation is regarded as a major cross-cutting issue in the PRSPs. In only 16 per cent of the Papers are young people seen as a group requiring integrated interventions. This, arguably, is the most important indicator of whether a PRSP addresses youth issues in a comprehensive manner. Piecemeal or single programme interventions are not likely to deliver the range of benefits an integrated approach can. The failure of just under half of the Governments to make use of feedback from young people in the preparation of the PRSPs is one likely cause of the piecemeal nature of most of the policy options adopted. The absence of accounts of young people experiencing poverty is a telling indicator of the lack of priority attached to youth as a distinct group in this context. What all of this means is that concerted, multisectoral government efforts to address their situation are unlikely.

Why are young people overlooked in poverty assessments?

One reason young people are overlooked in poverty assessments is that they are not viewed by authorities as economic or social dependants in the same way children are. Another reason may have to do with how data on the poor are collected. The methodology for compiling data on poverty defined from a dynamic perspective is far more complex than that used to collect data on poverty as a static condition.[1] For Governments espousing the dynamic view of poverty, aggregate cross-sectional data are insufficient; information must also be accumulated over time about the same individuals' or same groups' experiences of poverty. Most poverty assessments, such as those used in the formulation of PRSPs, rely on household surveys to identify the poor. These surveys usually focus on easily enumerated households, with each household comprising a dwelling and a family. Young people in poverty are likely to be underrepresented in such a context if they have left the parental home and are in precarious circumstances, perhaps living in temporary accommodations or in no accommodations at all.

When addressing poverty as a dynamic phenomenon, it is useful to construct risk profiles for different groups of poor people by measuring vulnerabilities. As articulated in the United Nations *Report on the World Social Situation, 2003*, vulnerability and poverty reinforce each other in a vicious circle. No social group is inherently vulnerable, but all groups experience specific vulnerabilities as a consequence of economic, social and cultural barriers (United Nations, 2003). Measuring vulnerabilities requires more than observing households on a one-time basis. Quite often, only data collected over time can produce the basic information needed to quantify the "volatility and vulnerability that poor households say is so important" (World Bank, 2001). Single-observation survey data cannot be used to track people's movements in and out of poverty and therefore cannot be used to identify vulnerabilities; "the challenge is to find indicators of vulnerability that can identify at-risk households and populations beforehand" (World Bank, 2001, p. 19).

THE VALUE OF ESTIMATING POVERTY AMONG YOUTH AT A NATIONAL LEVEL

Why is it worthwhile to derive estimates of young people in poverty at the national level? Performance indicators are usually developed with a particular audience and political purpose in mind. The extent to which specific targets serve as spurs to action will depend on how well they are incorporated by Governments into current national poverty reduction strategies and adopted by government agencies and other stakeholders such as NGOs in their immediate-term action plans.

Broad estimates of the numbers of poor youth at the global level have some value, as they indicate to international agencies and donors that poverty does not merely afflict children, families and older persons. However, it is at the country level that the estimates of young people in extreme poverty have the greatest impact, because this is the level at which public policy is usually formulated. A focus on young people is especially important in situations in which a national poverty reduction strategy has been or is about to be put in place.

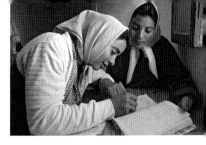

The first MDG has been criticized for its failure to define the specific reference group. The first target, which is to halve, by the year 2015, the proportion of the world's population whose income is less than US$ 1 a day, could apply at a national, regional or global level. For various reasons, the United Nations urges countries to interpret the MDGs as country-level goals (Pangestu and Sachs, 2004). One reason is that global measures do not guide policy. It is likely that the poverty target will be met on the basis of existing positive trends in China and India alone. However, to declare this a victory would be to disregard the millions of people living in extreme poverty in other parts of Asia and in Latin America and sub-Saharan Africa. Second, while a regional focus for the MDGs may highlight the needs of groups of countries with common characteristics, and may direct attention to the need for a coordinated response on the part of international agencies and donors, it may also prevent the performance of policymakers in individual countries from being scrutinized as closely as it should be. The third reason is that the country level represents "the greatest source of traction for poverty reduction. ... (C)ountries will only achieve the MDGs when national Governments are committed to making the necessary social investments in their citizens and when they receive adequate support to do so from the international system" (Pangestu and Sachs, 2004, p. 7).

The MDGs may seem ambitious for many of the poorest countries, but the fact is that every country in the world can achieve them within the next 10 years if intensive efforts are made by all parties (United Nations Millennium Project, 2005). The United Nations has encouraged countries to adopt and implement national development strategies "bold enough to meet the Millennium Development Goals targets for 2015" (United Nations, 2005a). Individual countries around the world have shown that it is possible, in a very short period of time, to dramatically reduce poverty while making enormous strides in advancing education, gender equality and other aspects of development. Official development assistance from the wealthier countries must be substantially increased, however, if the MDGs are to be achieved in the poorest countries (United Nations, 2005a).

For the reasons cited above, the following presentation of poverty data on young people focuses on individual countries. The value of such data is that they allow cross-country comparisons and raise questions about why some countries are doing better or worse than others. Unless the changing circumstances of young people in poverty are researched and the findings are presented in national forums, policymakers may continue to assign low priority to the specific needs of poor young people.

HEADCOUNT OF YOUNG PEOPLE IN EXTREME POVERTY

It is possible to use the widely accepted indicators of absolute income poverty to estimate the numbers of young people in extreme poverty. The proportion of people in a country living below the poverty line of US$ 1 or US$ 2 per person per day is adjusted based on the proportion of young people (aged 15-24 years) in the overall population; this simple calculation provides an indication of the number of youth who live below the poverty line.[2] Estimates of young people in poverty can be derived for countries for which there are no poverty measures by matching them with the closest country with an available poverty measure.[3]

Based on the most recent data available up to 2002, it is estimated that there are some 209 million young people living on less than US$ 1 a day and around 515 million young people living on less than US$ 2 a day (*see table 2.2*). These estimates have been derived from data provided in the World Bank's *World Development Indicators, 2004* on the proportions of people in each country living below the international poverty lines. The overall figures indicate that almost one in five young people (18 per cent of the 1,158 million 15- to 24-year olds worldwide) are living on less than US$ 1 per day,[4] while almost half (45 per cent) are living on less than US$ 2 per day.

Table 2.2
Regional estimates of young people* living in extreme poverty, 2002 (*Millions*)

Region	Numbers of young people living on less than US$ 1 per day	Numbers of young people living on less than US$ 2 per day
South Asia	84.1	206.1
East Asia and the Pacific	46.5	150.5
Sub-Saharan Africa	60.7	102.1
Latin America and the Caribbean	11.1	27.2
Europe and Central Asia	4.1	18.2
Middle East and North Africa	2.0	12.1
Total**	208.6	515.1

Source: The two sets of figures are calculated from data contained in the World Bank's World Development Indicators, 2004 on the proportion of people in each country living below the international poverty line (United Nations population estimates for 2000, derived from *World Population Prospects: The 2004 Revision, Population Database* (available from http://esa.un.org/unpp/)).

* Individuals between the ages of 15 and 24.

** Totals may not add precisely due to rounding.

The largest proportion of the world's poorest youth can be found in South Asia, which accounts for 4 out of every 10 young people living on less than US$ 1 or US$ 2 a day. Sub-Saharan Africa is home to 3 in 10 young people living on less than US$ 1 per day, and to 2 in 10 youth living on less than US$ 2 per day.

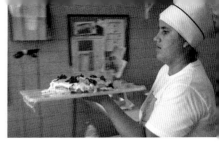

The 10 countries with the largest concentrations of young people living on less than US$ 1 a day are India (67.7 million), China (33.3 million), Nigeria (18.6 million), Bangladesh (9.9 million), Democratic Republic of the Congo (6.9 million), Pakistan (3.8 million), Sudan (3.7 million), Ethiopia (3.4 million), Indonesia (3.1 million) and Viet Nam (2.9 million). The list of countries with the largest concentrations of young people living on less than US$ 2 a day is the same, with one exception; Brazil replaces Sudan in tenth place. The ranking of countries is also slightly different, with Indonesia and Viet Nam moving up to the fifth and eighth positions respectively.

As noted earlier, sex-disaggregated indicators for per capita income are not available. However, the indicators used for other MDGs—relating to literacy, access to primary and secondary schooling, and access to health services—clearly show that girls and young women are much more likely than boys and young men to be disadvantaged (Curtain, 2004), though there may be significant intraregional variations. In South Asia, for example, the primary net enrolment ratio (females as a percentage of males enrolled in primary education) is lowest in Pakistan (55 per cent), followed by India (77 per cent) and Nepal (79 per cent), but Bangladesh and Sri Lanka have been able to achieve much better ratios (96 and 94 per cent respectively) (Curtain, 2004).

Changes over time?

The more recent global estimates of youth in extreme poverty can be compared with the estimates of 238 million and 462 million young people living on less than US$ 1 and US$ 2 a day, respectively, in the *World Youth Report, 2003*. The latter estimates were based on the international poverty lines reported in the World Development Indicators for 2000. The two sets of statistics suggest that the number of young people living on less than US$ 1 a day has decreased by nearly 30 million; it is likely, however, that a significant portion of this group has moved into the nominally better category of those living on less than US$ 2 per day, which has increased by 53 million.

Comparing estimates of young people in poverty over time is fraught with difficulties. The international poverty line measures are extrapolations from nationally representative household surveys, which constitute the primary sources of data. These surveys were undertaken in different years, and many are not recent. Some date from as far back as 1989 (Sierra Leone) and 1990/91 (Zimbabwe). Only two of the household surveys took place as recently as 2002 (Albania and Indonesia), and 10 include data for 2001 only. For the remaining 139 countries, the survey dates and periods of coverage fall between the early 1990s and the year 2000. As the source data used in the *World Development Indicators* are unlikely to change over a short time span for many countries, a meaningful comparison between two recent periods is difficult, if not impossible.

The use of poverty lines (such as the benchmark of US$ 1 a day) has been criticized in academic literature and policy discourse. One critique is that the poverty lines do not account for purchasing power differences between countries (Sala-i-Martin, 2002); a second is that the poverty lines are not based on the costing of the basic resource requirements; and a third relates to the uncertain baseline data on which the poverty estimates are based (Pogge and Reddy, 2003). Despite these observations, it may be argued that the current income poverty indicators do serve as an entry point for international comparisons of young people living in poverty.

National poverty lines

While the income poverty lines of US$ 1 and US$ 2 a day are useful for drawing international comparisons, nationally derived poverty measures are of much greater value for national policy purposes. National poverty estimates make it possible to derive subnational estimates, which are essential for targeting intracountry poverty reduction efforts. It is important to use national measures to determine the rates of poverty among young people; however, the substantial variation in household survey dates suggests that many countries are not undertaking regular surveys. In some cases this may be due to the lack of resources, though in other cases it may reflect a lack of political will to identify more specifically who the poor are and where young people stand in terms of national income distribution.

RURAL POVERTY

In many countries, poverty rates are substantially higher in rural areas than in urban areas. Some may argue that the rural-urban poverty gap is to some extent a statistical artefact— the result of shifts in urban boundaries as wealthier villages situated near towns are in time redefined as urban areas (Pogge and Reddy, 2003). Nonetheless, the fact remains that most poverty in developing countries occurs in rural areas and is especially prevalent among small farmers and landless families. Much of the poverty found in urban areas is a consequence of rural deprivation and rural economic decline, which trigger distress migration to the cities. In 1995, the United Nations General Assembly placed strong emphasis on rural development in the World Programme of Action for Youth, calling for actions focused on making farming more rewarding and life in rural areas more attractive for young people. Over the past 10 years, however, there has been a sharp decline in the national and international resources devoted to agricultural and rural development in developing countries (Food and Agriculture Organization of the United Nations, 2002; Majid, 2004). Poverty reduction efforts need to incorporate explicit agricultural growth strategies.

Rural youth should constitute a primary focus of interventions aimed at reducing poverty in order to stem the large-scale migration of young people to urban areas. Commitments made in the World Programme of Action for Youth in this regard should be implemented, supported by agricultural credit schemes for young people. Educational curricula should be adapted to address the needs of rural youth and enhance their skills. It should be noted, however, that these measures will meet with little success unless the agriculture sector undergoes a structural transformation at the global level, with particular attention given to facilitating market access and sharing new technologies.

YOUNG PEOPLE IN HUNGER

An alternative to the income measure of extreme poverty among young people is a measure based on levels of food energy intake. The Food and Agriculture Organization of the United Nations (FAO) estimates the prevalence of undernourishment at the country level by calculating the amount of food available per person and the extent of inequality in access to food (Food and Agriculture Organization of the United Nations, 2003). The value of this approach is that it uses a common energy measure (kilocalorie intake) and is therefore potentially comparable across countries.

FAO has been criticized for basing its measure on country-level estimates of annual food supplies derived from data on production, imports, exports, changes in stock, and supply utilization summarized in food balance sheets. In contrast, the countries themselves derive estimates of dietary energy consumption from household expenditure surveys and/or household food consumption surveys (David, 2002).[5] FAO has defended its method as the "only way currently available to arrive at global and regional estimates of the prevalence of undernourishment" (Food and Agriculture Organization of the United Nations, 2003, p. 6). However, a 2002 symposium of experts called for efforts to improve both the data and the analytical approach used to derive these estimates (Food and Agriculture Organization of the United Nations, 2003).

Table 2.3 presents estimates of the numbers of undernourished young people in the major regions and worldwide. The figures are derived from FAO country estimates of undernourishment for the total population, averaged over the period 1999-2001. The estimated total of 160.1 million undernourished young people is lower than the income poverty estimate of 209 million young people living on less than US$ 1 per day.

The regional distributions in table 2.3 show that South Asia accounts for the largest number of undernourished young people, with the highest concentrations found in Bangladesh, India and Pakistan. Sub-Saharan Africa is next, with the highest national concentrations found in the Democratic Republic of the Congo, Ethiopia, Kenya, Mozambique, Nigeria and South Africa. East Asia and the Pacific has the third-highest number of undernourished young people.

Table 2.3
Regional and global estimates of undernourished young people,*
1999-2001

Region	Number of young people undernourished (in millions)	Undernourished youth as a percentage of the global total
South Asia	57.8	36.1
Sub-Saharan Africa	39.9	24.9
East Asia and the Pacific	38.6	24.1
Latin America and the Caribbean	10.8	6.8
Middle East and North Africa	7.1	4.4
Europe and Central Asia	5.8	3.6
Total**	160.1	100

Sources: UNDP, *Human Development Report, 2004: Cultural Liberty in Today's Diverse World* (United Nations publication, Sales No. E.04.III.B.1), table 7; and United Nations population estimates for 2000, derived from *World Population Prospects: The 2004 Revision, Population Database* (available from http://esa.un.org/unpp/)).
    * Individuals between the ages of 15 and 24.
    ** Totals may not add precisely due to rounding.

POLICIES AND PROGRAMMES
FOR POVERTY ALLEVIATION

There is no single recipe for alleviating poverty among youth. Poverty eradication measures are as numerous and varied as the causes of poverty. Successful country-level strategies reflect an integrated approach based on local, regional and national assessments of the range of problems poor young people face. This integrated approach should be applied in national pro-poor growth strategies, with specific provisions for infrastructure development and agricultural policy changes that will benefit the poor. Youth-focused strategies will be most effective if young people are involved in their design and implementation.

A paper entitled "Investing in children and youth for poverty reduction" outlines the various types of public investment that may be undertaken to reduce poverty among young people in the age group 12-25 (Hoddinott and Quisumbing, 2003). The suggested measures, listed separately according to whether the investments are directly or indirectly aimed at young people, are displayed in table 2.4.

Table 2.4
Suggested forms of public action aimed at improving the situation of adolescents and young people

Direct Measures	Indirect Measures
Employment/sporadic unemployment	Long-term unemployment
<ul><li>Improved public provision of secondary education</li><li>Improved design and quality of education service delivery, measures for girls to continue to secondary school</li><li>Scholarship programmes for girls</li><li>Basic education and literacy training for adolescents</li><li>Conditional cash transfer programmes</li><li>Reproductive health-care and peer counselling</li><li>Programmes to reduce tobacco consumption</li><li>On-the-job training and work-study programmes</li><li>Tertiary education</li></ul>	<ul><li>Time-saving infrastructure</li><li>Labour regulations that do not reduce employment</li><li>Macro policies conducive to employment and distribution-oriented growth</li><li>Infrastructure development to create a favourable business environment</li><li>Labour market laws that do not discriminate against women</li></ul>

Source: J. Hoddinott and A. Quisumbing, "Investing in children and youth for poverty reduction" (Washington, D.C., International Food Policy Research Institute, 24 June 2003), p. 24.

At both the national and international levels, the successful elements of relevant policies and programmes must be identified and scaled up if they are to have any real impact on poverty reduction (also see chapter 1, section 3). Many countries have youth policies and/or youth development programmes in place. Few of the existing youth programmes have been evaluated for their effectiveness, however, which means that information about successful investments in youth is lacking. Where reliable indications of effectiveness exist, progress has been measured over too short a period to allow meaningful assessment (Curtain, 2004).

CONCLUSION

This chapter has advanced the argument that a reduction in absolute poverty should serve as the primary test of whether a country's growth strategy is successful. This line of reasoning requires that national poverty reduction strategies constitute an integral part of national development strategies. In developing national strategies for poverty reduction, special attention should be focused on the needs of particular groups of young people who have been excluded from opportunities to benefit from economic growth.

The income- and hunger-based estimates presented in this chapter highlight the regional and global magnitude of poverty among youth. Young people living in poverty will not be given the attention they deserve in national poverty reduction strategies until their situation is formally acknowledged, they are properly consulted, and appropriate information is obtained on the nature and extent of their vulnerabilities.

Although there is some dispute over the reliability and universal applicability of the international poverty line and the FAO methodology for estimating the number of undernourished people in the world, these income- and energy-based measures offer some indication of the vast numbers of young people affected. The global estimates presented in the chapter suggest that 160 million young people are experiencing extreme hunger, 209 million young people are living on less than US$ 1 a day, and 515 million young people are living on less than US$ 2 a day. It is also noted that poverty is most prevalent in rural areas.

The targets specified in the MDGs will not be met by 2015 unless countries adopt a broad range of public policies aimed at addressing all forms and aspects of poverty. Some policymakers continue to view economic growth as a panacea for reducing poverty, with little attention given to the need for country-specific strategies that reflect a more dynamic view of poverty. The PRSP process represents an attempt to promote the development of tailor-made strategies for poverty reduction; however, the Papers that have been produced thus far have been criticized for appearing strikingly similar, even for countries that face very different challenges (Vandemoortele, 2004). It may be inferred that these national poverty reduction strategies are in many cases not genuinely "home-grown".

While little is known about the specific characteristics of young people in poverty, it has been possible in this chapter to make the case for targeted interventions aimed at youth development. Young people account for a large share of the population in most countries. Societies that fail to acknowledge the particular challenges facing youth and to involve them in devising solutions will find it difficult to achieve the MDGs, including sharp reductions in poverty levels, by 2015. Addressing the health, education and employment needs of young people can contribute to economic growth, generating additional income for both individuals and Governments that may, in turn, be used for human development. Investing in youth can therefore initiate a virtuous cycle of pro-poor development. The price that countries pay for not investing in youth development may be economic decline and rising poverty.

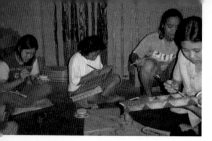

Young people in extreme poverty represent a special challenge for those tasked with developing home-grown poverty reduction strategies. Existing research may be overly focused on groups living in chronic poverty. Many young people are more likely to experience a less static form, moving in and out of poverty. The transition from childhood to adulthood involves confronting and overcoming a number of uncertainties. Young people may also experience a series of major changes during this period, compounding any difficulties they may face, including challenges relating to employment, living arrangements, personal relationships, or socio-economic status. Identifying the uncertainties and potential outcomes faced by young people or subgroups of young people is the first step in devising ways to improve levels of social protection. Sets of regularly updated indicators, presented in the form a youth development index, could prove useful in evaluating the social and economic circumstances of youth and the changes that occur over time.

Governments, donors and civil society organizations must be guided by a comprehensive national perspective in their efforts to address poverty among young people. A network of major stakeholders must be established to ensure the coordination of efforts across government departments and the donor community. Extensive, ongoing consultation with young people and their representative associations is required at all stages of the policy development and implementation process.

Direct primary information and evidence is a crucial input in the policymaking process, especially in relation to young people. Consideration must be given to the particular situations faced by specific groups of youth as a consequence of factors such as gender, race, rural or urban residence, and the stage of the life cycle. Finally, once the key elements of a national poverty reduction strategy (including youth-targeted policies and activities) have been identified, the challenge is to work out ways to scale up the essential features of successful initiatives so that they can have a major impact on poverty reduction. ●

---

[1] The World Bank's *World Development Report, 2000/2001* notes that "measuring vulnerability is especially difficult: since the concept is dynamic, it cannot be measured merely by observing households once. Only with household panel data—that is, household surveys that follow the same households over several years—can the basic information be gathered to capture and quantify the volatility and vulnerability that poor households say is so important. Moreover, people's movements in and out of poverty are informative about vulnerability only after the fact. The challenge is to find indicators of vulnerability that can identify at-risk households and populations beforehand." (World Bank, 2001, p. 19)

[2] The assumption is that young people are likely to experience poverty no less or no more than the population as a whole.

[3] This method is similar to the one used by Bourguignon and Morrisson (2002).

[4] Total population figures for young people are based on United Nations data (United Nations, 2005b).

[5] David also notes that "FAO's continued reliance on energy supply derived from national food balance sheets instead of energy consumption estimated from household sample surveys results in lack of coherence between the agency's estimates and those of the countries. Since there are no sub-national food balance sheets compilations in general, the FAO methodology cannot produce estimates at these levels. And the continued production of the FAO estimates in Rome does not engender the countries' collaboration or use of the indicators." (David, 2002, p. 17)

Bibliography

Bourguignon, F., and C. Morrisson (2002). Inequality among world citizens: 1820-1992. *The American Economic Review*, vol. 92, No. 4 (September), pp. 727-744.

Brown, B., and R. Larson (2002). The kaleidoscope of adolescence: experiences of the world's youth at the beginning of the 21st century. In *The World's Youth: Adolescence in Eight Regions of the Globe*, B. Bradford Brown, Reed W. Larson and T.S. Saraswathi, eds. Cambridge, United Kingdom: Cambridge University Press.

Curtain, R. (2004). The case for investing in young people as part of a national poverty reduction strategy. Paper commissioned by the United Nations Population Fund for the Technical Meeting on Promoting Sexual and Reproductive Health and Reproductive Rights: Reducing Poverty and Achieving the MDGs, Stockholm, 5-6 October, pp. 22-32 and 34.

David, I. (2002). On comparability of poverty statistics from different sources and disaggregation levels. Paper prepared for the United Nations Economic and Social Commission for Asia and the Pacific Committee on Statistics at its thirteenth session, Bangkok, 27-29 November.

Food and Agriculture Organization of the United Nations (2003). *The State of Food Insecurity in the World, 2003: Monitoring Progress towards the World Food Summit and Millennium Development Goals*. Rome.

_____, International Fund for Agricultural Development and World Food Programme (2002). Reducing poverty and hunger: the critical role of financing for food, agriculture and rural development. Paper prepared for the International Conference on Financing for Development, Monterrey, Mexico, 18-22 March. Rome: Food and Agriculture Organization of the United Nations.

Hoddinott, J., and A. Quisumbing (2003). Investing in children and youth for poverty reduction. Washington, D.C.: International Food Policy Research Institute, June 24.

Hulme, D., and A. Shepherd (2003). Conceptualizing chronic poverty. *World Development*, vol. 31, No. 3 (March).

International Labour Organization (2003). Working out of poverty. Report of the Director General presented to the International Labour Conference at its 91st session. Geneva.

Joint United Nations Programme on HIV/AIDS (2004). *2004 Report on the Global AIDS Epidemic: 4th Global Report*. Geneva.

Majid, N. (2004). Reaching Millennium Goals: How well does agricultural productivity growth reduce poverty? Geneva: International Labour Organization.

Mozambique (2001). *Action Plan for the Reduction of Absolute Poverty (2001-2005)*. Maputo.

Pangestu, M., and J. Sachs, coordinators (2004). *Interim Report of Task Force 1 on Poverty and Economic Development*. New York: United Nations Development Programme. 10 February.

Pernia, E. (2003). Pro-poor growth: what is it and how is it important? Economic Research Department Policy Brief No. 17. Manila: Asian Development Bank.

Pogge, T., and S. Reddy (2003). Unknown: the extent, distribution, and trend of global income poverty. New York: Columbia University/Institute of Social Analysis.

Rosen, J. (2003). *Adolescent Health and Development: A Resource Guide for World Bank Staff and Government Counterparts*. Washington, D.C.: World Bank

Sala-i-Martin, X. (2002). The disturbing "rise" of global income inequality. NBER Working Paper No. 8904 (April). Cambridge, Massachusetts: National Bureau of Economic Research.

United Nations (2003). *Report on the World Social Situation, 2003 — Social Vulnerability: Sources and Challenges*. Sales No. E.03.IV.10.

_____ (2005a). In larger freedom: towards development, security and human rights for all; report of the Secretary-General. A/59/2005. 21 March.

_____ (2005b). *World Population Prospects: The 2004 Revision*. ST/ESA/SER.A/244.

United Nations Development Programme (various years). *Human Development Report.* New York: Oxford University Press.

United Nations Millennium Project (2005). *Investing in Development: A Practical Plan to Achieve the Millennium Development Goals.* New York: United Nations Development Programme.

United Nations Population Fund (2004). *State of the World Population, 2004 — The Cairo Consensus at Ten: Population, Reproductive Health and the Global Effort to End Poverty.* New York.

Vandemoortele, J. (2004). Can the MDGs foster a new partnership for pro-poor policies? New York: United Nations Development Programme.

Waiselfisz, J.J. (2004). *Youth Development Report, 2003.* Brasilia: Office of the United Nations Educational, Scientific and Cultural Organization in Brazil (UNESCO Brasil).

Wood, G. (2003). Staying secure, staying poor: the "Faustian bargain". *World Development*, vol. 31, No. 3 (March), pp. 455-471.

World Bank (2001). *World Development Report, 2000/2001: Attacking Poverty.* Washington, D.C., and New York: World Bank and Oxford University Press.

_____ (2004). Sharpening the focus on poverty reduction. In *World Bank Development Report, 2005: A Better Investment Climate for Everyone.* Washington, D.C., and New York: World Bank and Oxford University Press.

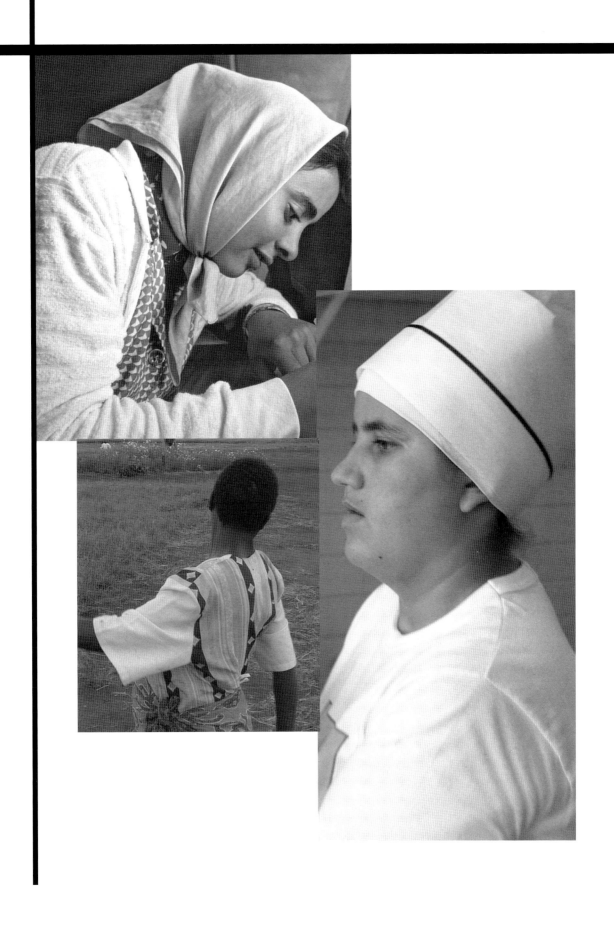

Chapter 3

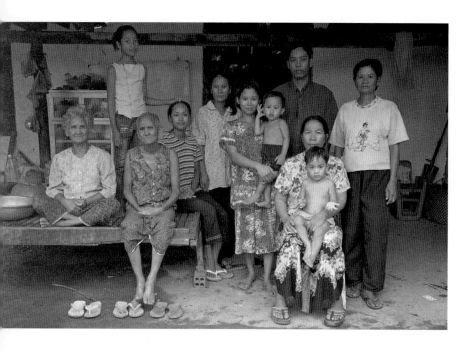

Chronic,
life-course
&
intergenerational poverty

The present chapter comprises a review of the related concepts of chronic poverty, life-course poverty and intergenerational poverty, and argues that these concepts contribute to a better understanding of youth poverty. The argument is elucidated and further developed through empirical data.

In the first part of the chapter, this argument is supported by evidence showing that much youth poverty has its roots in childhood poverty, and that some childhood poverty has its roots in youth poverty. In reference to the first point, it has been shown that the poverty experienced by youth is often linked to childhood deprivation and parental[1] poverty; essentially, the older generation has been unable to provide the assets the younger generation requires to overcome the challenges arising during youth. These challenges may be both structural and idiosyncratic. As to the second point, like poverty in childhood or in old age, poverty during youth can have implications for both an individual's life course and that of his or her household. In many cases, children born to youth in poverty may be especially susceptible to persistent poverty.

Drawing on these two main points, the second part of the chapter presents estimates of youth in extreme poverty based on a new child-centred approach to estimating childhood deprivation.[2] The third part assesses the policy implications of the findings and conclusions highlighted in this chapter.

THE RELEVANCE OF CHRONIC, LIFE-COURSE AND INTERGENERATIONAL POVERTY TO YOUTH POVERTY
The chronic poor

It is estimated that between 300 million and 420 million people are trapped in chronic, or persistent, poverty (Chronic Poverty Research Centre, 2004). Chronically poor people experience deprivation over many years, often over their entire lives, and sometimes pass poverty on to their children. Many of the chronically poor die prematurely from health problems that are easily preventable. This group experiences deprivation at multiple levels; chronic poverty is typically characterized not only by low income and assets, but also by hunger and undernutrition, illiteracy, the lack of access to basic necessities such as safe drinking water and health services, and social isolation and exploitation.

The chronically poor are not a distinct group but are typically those experiencing discrimination, stigmatization or "invisibility", including socially marginalized ethnic, religious, indigenous, nomadic and caste groups; migrants and bonded labourers; refugees and internally displaced persons; and people with disabilities and certain illnesses such as HIV/AIDS. In many contexts, poor women and girls, children, and older people (especially widows) are more likely to be trapped in poverty.

While chronically poor people are found in all parts of the world, the largest number (134 million to 188 million) live in South Asia. Sub-Saharan Africa has the highest prevalence, with 30 to 40 per cent of all those living on less than US$ 1 per day (an estimated 90 million to 120 million people) trapped in chronic poverty. East Asia has between 54 million and 85 million chronically poor people, most of whom live in China.

Within countries, chronic poverty tends to occur more frequently in certain geographical contexts. Higher concentrations of the chronically poor are often found in remote and low-potential rural settings, politically marginalized regions, and areas that are not well connected to markets, ports or urban centres—places that are often home to indigenous communities. There are also concentrations of chronically poor people in the slums of towns and cities, and millions are homeless.

The causes of chronic poverty are complex and highly variable. They may be the same as the causes of poverty, only more intense, widespread and lasting. In other cases, there is a qualitative difference between the causes of transitory poverty and the causes of chronic poverty. Rarely is there a single, clear cause. Chronic poverty usually derives from the confluence or overlap of multiple factors operating within contexts ranging from the household to the global milieu.[3] Some of these factors are "maintainers" of chronic poverty and serve to keep poor people poor. Others are "drivers" of chronic poverty; they push vulnerable non-poor and transitorily poor people into a deeper and more tenacious form of poverty from which they cannot escape. Not all chronically poor people are born into long-term deprivation. Many slide into chronic poverty after a shock or series of shocks from which they are unable to recover. Shocks experienced during particular periods in the life course of an individual or household, including adolescence or young adulthood, can be particularly damaging in this respect. Figure 3.1 outlines the key drivers of chronic poverty, with a focus on the implications of the different processes for youth.

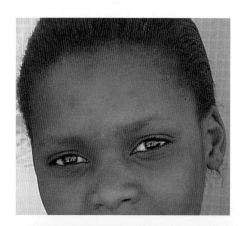
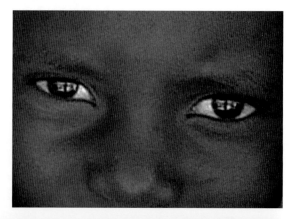
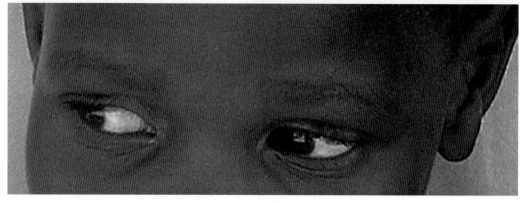

Figure 3.1
The main drivers of chronic poverty and their implications for young people

Key drivers of chronic poverty	Examples of implications for youth
Severe and/or repeated shocks	
• Ill health and injury	
• Environmental shocks and natural disasters	
• Market and economic collapse	
• Violence and conflict	
• Breakdown of law and order	

PLUS

Few private or collective assets to fall back on	Young people are often in the early stages of physical and financial asset accumulation and may find it especially difficult to weather and bounce back from shocks.
• Limited physical, financial, social or human capital; highly susceptible to shocks	

PLUS

Ineffective institutional support	Young couples may deplete their assets or reduce their own consumption to ensure that their young children receive health care or education where these services are costly. Even in labour markets with social insurance and other protective mechanisms in place, young people generally have not built up the time or contributions to benefit.
• The lack of effective social protection, public information, basic services, and conflict prevention and resolution	

PLUS

PLUS

Poverty occurring at certain points in an individual's or household's life course	When a young person is forced to discontinue his or her studies before completing the full secondary, tertiary or vocational course, there are reduced returns on, or a complete loss of, the significant long-term time and resource investments in education made by the young person and his or her family. It becomes more difficult to find productive work and rebuild assets.
• For example, in utero; during childhood, old age or youth; or among young households (*see column 2*)	

LIKELY TO TRAP PEOPLE IN POVERTY

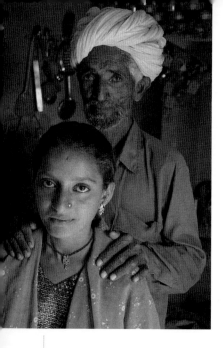

Six key maintainers of chronic poverty have been identified as well:[4]

- *No, low or narrow-based economic growth* provides few opportunities for poor people to raise their incomes and accumulate assets. The employment effects of such growth scenarios appear to be most extreme for youth. In the majority of countries, young people are two to four times more likely than those over the age of 25 to be unemployed (International Labour Organization, 2004). This may be at least partially attributable to the real or perceived lower skill levels and more limited social capital networks among youth (Save the Children/Childhood Poverty Research and Policy Centre, 2004). Young people who have the requisite skills and education but are nonetheless unable to find or keep decent or productive work may experience disillusionment, disappointment and desperation, undermining their sense of well-being and making them more vulnerable to recruitment by militant groups or organized crime.[5]

- *The interaction of social exclusion and adverse incorporation* forces those who suffer discrimination and stigmatization to engage in economic activities and social relations that keep them poor. Such individuals often have low-paid jobs with no security, low and declining assets, and minimal access to social protection and basic services, and many are dependent on patrons. In a number of contexts, being young increases one's chances of experiencing discrimination, particularly in the labour market. Young people who also suffer other forms of discrimination based on gender, impairment or ethnic status, for example, will be particularly hard hit; such circumstances are not uncommon. Further, if young people have not had the opportunity to build their own networks, they will be entirely dependent on the social and political capital of their households and communities. Where the latter are weak or destructive, as is the case with client households and marginalized ethnic minority groups, the capacity of young people to build their own positive socio-political relationships may be limited.

- *The circumstances prevailing in disadvantaged geographical and agroecological regions* perpetuate chronic poverty. Poor natural resources, infrastructure and basic services; weak economic integration; and social exclusion and political marginality create "logjams of disadvantage". Youth are often particularly determined to escape remote, marginal, or economically stagnant areas, and some are able to migrate to urban areas and build better lives. However, limited skills and social networks, membership in an ethnic or linguistic minority, and a lack of access to information undermine the efforts of many young people to establish a sustaining urban livelihood. Those young people who are unable to migrate owing to factors such as gender, illness, impairment, family responsibilities and extreme deprivation can experience disappointment and desperation.

- *High and persistent capability deprivation*, especially during childhood — exemplified by poor nutrition, untreated illness, and the lack of access to education — diminishes human development in ways that are often irreversible. Pregnant women who suffered poor health and nutrition during their own childhood and adolescence face a higher risk of maternal and child mortality and morbidity, and early childbearing compounds the risk. It has been estimated that in 2004, 17 per cent of all births in least developed countries occurred among women aged 15-19 years. The babies born to these young mothers are at greater risk of ill-health. Unhealthy, poorly educated children can grow into young people with limited capacities for learning and working. However, adolescence and young adulthood, when individuals are learning how to function more independently, may constitute a window of opportunity. Improvements in skills, education, health and nutritional status during these periods may override earlier disadvantages (*also see figure 3.4 and the subsequent tex*t).

- *In weak, failing or failed States*, where economic opportunities are few and basic services and social protection are lacking, people can easily fall into desperate poverty, and the inadequacy of official support mechanisms and the powerlessness of the poor themselves make it unlikely that they will secure their rights and escape poverty.

- *Weak or failed international cooperation* can lead to a dramatic increase in the incidence of chronic poverty. In the 1980s and 1990s, structural adjustment policies and programmes and rapid economic liberalization negatively affected economic growth and employment, aid allocations, and trade opportunities for many countries with large numbers of chronically poor people, deepening poverty in many cases.

The knowledge now available about chronic poverty must be used to mobilize public action and reshape development strategies. While there are many policies that are potentially beneficial for both the poor and the chronically poor, many people living in chronic poverty are not "just like the poor, but (are) further down the poverty spectrum" (Chronic Poverty Research Centre, 2004). Overcoming chronic poverty requires policymakers to reorder their priorities and set their sights higher than the current policy consensus on poverty reduction. Development strategies need to move beyond the current emphasis on economic growth; hundreds of millions of people are born poor, live poor and die poor in the midst of increasing wealth. Chronically poor people need more than opportunities to improve their situation. They require targeted support and protection, as well as political action to deal with the problem of exclusion. If policymakers wish to open the door to genuine development for chronically poor people, they must first address the inequality, discrimination and exploitation that drive and maintain chronic poverty. Actions that may be taken to alleviate chronic, intergenerational and youth poverty will be detailed later in this chapter.

Poverty dynamics

Dealing with chronic poverty requires an understanding of poverty dynamics—the changes in well-being or ill-being that individuals and households experience over time. Falling into poverty, remaining stuck in poverty, and escaping poverty are the products of different combinations of structural and idiosyncratic factors operating at the individual, household, community, national and global levels. Life-course events, including transitions into adulthood and old age, marriage and having children, and the loss of a spouse, may seriously affect a person's vulnerability to poverty.

Conventional analysis is based on poverty trends, which reflect changes in poverty rates at the aggregate level. This approach offers no details about important processes and particular circumstances at the household level. Information on the progress achieved in Viet Nam can be used to illustrate this point. During the 1990s, the country experienced a remarkable reduction in poverty; from 1993 to 1998, rural and urban poverty rates fell by about 24 and 15 per cent respectively. However, these aggregate poverty trends provide no indication of what occurred among individual households. In rural areas, one third of the population remained poor, and another 5 per cent fell into poverty (*see figure 3.2a*). The urban picture is nowhere near as disheartening; about 7 per cent stayed in poverty, while only about 2 per cent moved into poverty (*see figure 3.2b*). Why did over half of the rural poor and more than one quarter of the urban poor fail to benefit from the country's pro-poor growth strategies? More detailed, focused data can provide a clearer picture-indicating, for example, that in the urban areas of Viet Nam the chronically poor are more likely to be wage workers, while in rural areas they rely on subsistence agriculture; and that children in chronically poor households are much more likely to be undernourished or malnourished and out of school.

Figure 3.2a
Poverty dynamics in rural
Viet Nam, 1993-1998

Figure 3.2b
Poverty dynamics in urban
Viet Nam, 1993-1998

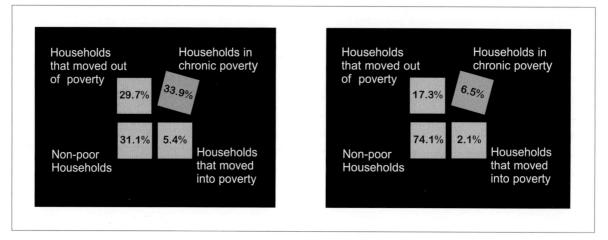

Source: B. Baulch, based on the Viet Nam Living Standards Survey panel, in the *Chronic Poverty Report, 2004-05* (Manchester, Institute for Development Policy and Management/Chronic Poverty Research Centre, 2004).

An understanding of poverty dynamics provides a sounder basis for anti-poverty policy formulation than reliance on poverty trends alone. Achieving a more nuanced understanding of poverty requires the collection of both panel data and standard cross-sectional household survey data. In cross-sectional household surveys, data are collected from a representative sample of households, but the same households are not necessarily included in each survey. In contrast, panel data are longitudinal data sets that track the same households over time. Ideally, panel data sets should be comprised of more than two waves of data collection so that households that are poor in every period (the chronically poor) can be distinguished from those that are poor in at least one but not all periods (the transitorily poor, who move in and out of poverty).

Conceptualizing and measuring poverty over the life course

The collection and analysis of panel data, as well as innovative qualitative inputs such as life histories, provide a clearer understanding of the ways in which the occurrence and experience of poverty can change across the life courses of individuals and households. At certain points or stages in the life course, poverty based on structural discrimination may be exacerbated and may become more deeply entrenched, and cross-sectional data do not provide much help in disentangling cohort effects from life-course effects.

This concept is best illustrated through an example that details the relevant data requirements and accompanying analytical processes. Data show, for instance, that women over the age of 65 are twice as likely to be living in poverty as adult women younger than 45 years of age. Using cross-sectional survey data alone, it would be difficult to determine whether this occurs primarily owing to a cohort effect, an example being that older women are less likely to be literate than their younger counterparts, who have grown up with different educational opportunities and gender roles; or to a life-course effect, based on the fact that women are more likely to be widowed, dependent and/or in ill-health as they age. As people get older, their roles, capacities and responsibilities change, as do the opportunities available to them. These shifts occur within the context of continuously evolving relationships and circumstances both within and outside the household. Changes in household composition (including size, dependency ratios[6] and headship) through marriage, divorce, abandonment, birth, illness, death, and migration have a differential impact on household members depending on their age, gender and health status; these are important considerations in assessing how poverty and well-being are experienced by individuals within such a context. Returning to the example, panel data can provide a better idea of whether education or other assets accumulated by younger cohorts will allow them to overcome the challenges thrown at them as they age.

In support of this argument, it is recommended to use panel data sets to measure the extent of youth poverty, as young people are more likely to be experiencing a more dynamic form of poverty due to the obstacles most face in seeking to achieve adult status (life-course effects) (United Nations Population Fund, 2005). It is intuitively understood that youth, however defined, are presented with an especially dynamic set of challenges and opportunities; as noted in the previous chapter, the transition from childhood to adulthood is characterized by major changes and involves confronting and overcoming a number of difficulties and uncertainties, including obstacles relating to employment, living arrangements, personal relationships, and socio-economic status.

It is this dynamism that makes "youth" so difficult to define in functional terms. The extent to which a young person is economically dependent, independent, or depended upon can change extremely rapidly, with significant implications for his or her present and long-term well-being. This is demonstrated in an example featuring four 18-year-old women living in urban Asia:

- Anna lives with her parents and siblings. She is in full-time education and does not work.

- Meena lives alone in a women's hostel and works in a garment factory. She supports herself and sends money to her parents in the village for her siblings' education.

- Sonia lives alone with her husband. She is a nursery school teacher and also works at home.

- Tania lives with her husband and two small children, her in-laws, and her father-in-law's parents. She works at home.

None of these women is unusual, yet even from this thumbnail sketch it is apparent that each has a very different set of roles and responsibilities, as well as different opportunities and resources that can be tapped during a crisis. Furthermore, within a very short period of time—perhaps three years—Anna can "become" Meena, then Sonia, then Tania. Responsibility for a young woman's well-being may shift from her parents to herself to her husband and in-laws, and she may assume a certain amount of responsibility for the needs of her own children and those of some of her siblings. She may find a particular set of socio-economic circumstances more or less challenging depending on, for example, how many dependants she has, the extent of her available resources, and whether she is allowed or forced to work outside the home. Regardless of her situation, she will still belong to the group defined as "youth".

Longitudinal data can help analysts determine how, why and to what extent poverty status and other indicators of well-being are affected by the changes and circumstances occurring during the transition from childhood to youth, through youth into adulthood, and throughout the life course. Exemplifying this process is a recent study from the United Kingdom of Great Britain and Northern Ireland that uses 10 waves of the British Household Panel Survey and combines longitudinal and cohort analysis of income trajectories for people at different stages of their lives to build a picture of income dynamics over the whole life cycle (Rigg and Sefton, 2004).

Importantly, the "life stages" identified in the study are not entirely age-dependent; in the model, having a partner and/or children of various ages makes a difference. While moving into, through or out of a specific life stage affects the likelihood of experiencing particular life events, age is not the only factor defining a particular stage. Furthermore, the

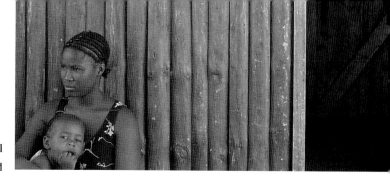

life stages are not sequential, can overlap, may not all be experienced by all people, or may be experienced more than once. Anna and Tania from the example above are the same age but at different stages in their lives, and this affects the likelihood of each young woman starting a job or becoming a widow, for example.

The study findings indicate that certain life events are closely associated with specific income trajectories in the United Kingdom; partnership formation and children becoming independent are associated with upward trajectories, while having children and retiring are associated with downward trajectories. However, there is considerable heterogeneity in income trajectories following these different events, and a downward trajectory does not equate to a slide into poverty. When age alone is considered, the results show that youth (older children and young adults aged 11-24 years) are relatively likely to experience an upward trajectory but also a higher proportion of unstable trajectories (Rigg and Sefton, 2004).

Long-term and well-analysed panel data sets are available for many high-income countries; however, panel data sets from low- and middle-income countries that allow analysis of poverty dynamics are few and far between. The nature and structure of longitudinal surveys are such that substantial funding is required for data collection and analysis over the long term, which tends to be incompatible with the budgetary cycles of government statistical offices or donor bodies. Those panels that do exist are often not nationally representative; they may be undertaken only in one region, or in rural but not urban areas, for example. All longitudinal data sets suffer from participant attrition and changes in definitions and topics of interest over time; this is especially true for cross-sectional household surveys that are later turned into panels. Furthermore, cross-country comparability is limited by the very different lengths of time between surveys, ranging from one to ten years. The majority of longitudinal studies span less than five years and/or include only two waves of data.[7] Most data sets are not accessible (or affordable) to researchers outside the host institutions.[8] Those sets with data sufficiently disaggregated to analyse poverty by age or life stage are even rarer.

Some recent developments indicate that the situation is beginning to change. There are currently two large-scale, child-focused longitudinal surveys under way in the developing world, one of which makes children's experiences of poverty the focus of analysis. Young Lives, initiated in 2001, is investigating changes in child poverty over a 15-year period in Ethiopia, India, Peru and Viet Nam. Birth to Twenty, initiated in 1990, explores the social, economic, political, demographic and nutrition-related transitions under way in urban South Africa and the impact of these changes on a cohort of children, adolescents and their families.

Several longitudinal survey projects have recently undertaken additional waves of data collection (for example, in Indonesia), while others are planning to do so (in Bangladesh and Mexico, for instance), and many intend to make the data sets publicly available within a reasonable amount of time.

In the previous chapter, it was argued that young people were less likely to be identified as a target group for poverty reduction in those countries in which a static view of poverty prevailed, given the tendency in such contexts to focus on persistent poverty among the long-term poor. Life-course factors are often not given adequate consideration in traditional poverty analysis; however, one could argue that while the features of youth poverty tend to be highly dynamic, young people can also experience chronic poverty. This is especially likely when youth poverty is grounded in parental and childhood poverty, and when it has implications for a youth's entire life course as well as that of his or her offspring. Longitudinal data are required to understand both aspects of youth poverty-the long-term causes and implications as well as the shorter-term fluctuations in opportunities, obstacles and well-being.[9]

The intergenerational transmission of poverty

A livelihood approach, focusing on transfers of assets or capital (or the absence thereof) in the context of social, institutional and policy environments, is useful for understanding the intergenerational transmission of poverty. There are two major factors contributing to this intergenerational dynamic: poverty may or may not be privately transmitted from older generations of individuals and families to younger generations (especially, but not exclusively, from parents to their children); and resources may or may not be publicly transferred from one generation to the next (an example is taxing the income of older generations to finance primary education). Transfers can be positive (cash assets, positive aspirations) or negative (bonded labour obligations, poor nutrition, gender discrimination). As shown in table 3.1, different kinds of assets may be transferred or not transferred through various modes and mechanisms, depending on the circumstances.

Source: Adapted from Karen Moore, "Frameworks for understanding the intergenerational transmission of poverty and well-being in developing countries", CPRC Working Paper No. 8 (Manchester, United Kingdom, Institute for Development Policy and Management/Chronic Poverty Research Centre, 2001).

* It is argued that "'cultures of poverty' exist based upon the ways in which the poor have adapted to and coped with poverty over years and generations. These values, beliefs and behaviours may have been useful and appropriate in the context of the structural impediments faced by earlier generations, but remain as obstacles to development among new generations although structures may have changed. The 'culture of poverty' becomes a poverty-related structure in itself." (O. Lewis, *Five Families: Mexican Case Studies in the Culture of Poverty* (NewYork, Basic Books, 1959), in K. Moore, "Frameworks for understanding the intergenerational transmission of poverty...", p. 14.)

Table 3.1
The livelihood approach to intergenerationally transmitted poverty

What is transmitted or not transmitted?	How is it transmitted or not transmitted?	Possible implications for youth
Financial, material and environmental capital		
• Cash • Land • Livestock • Housing, buildings • Other productive/non-productive physical assets • Common property resources • Debt	• Insurance, pensions • Inheritance, bequests, dispossession • Gifts, loans • Dowry, bride wealth • Environmental conservation/degradation • Labour bondage	• Depending on the socio-legal context, young women or men may not be able to access, own or manage particular forms of assets, including inherited assets, leaving them dependent on older relatives. • Dowry demands can affect recently married young women and their families in particular.
Human capital		
• Educational qualifications, knowledge, skills, coping/survival strategies • Good mental/physical health • Disease, impairment	• Socialization • Investment of time/capital in care; education/training; health/nutrition • Contagion, mother-to-child transmission • Genetic inheritance	• Youth are often expected to make a transition from full-time education to employment if they have not done so already, potentially affecting parental investment in education or training. • Youth and adults of working age account for a disproportionate share of those living with HIV/AIDS; this has negative short- and long-term implications for the sufferer, his or her household (especially children and older people), and the economy.
Social, cultural and political capital		
• Traditions, institutions, norms of entitlement, value systems • Position in the community • Access to key decision makers, patrons, organizations • "Cultures of poverty"?*	• Socialization and education • Kinship • Locality • Genetic inheritance	• Young people are often key targets for those attempting to build or maintain social, political or cultural movements. This can help determine what other forms of capital are available to them, as well as the livelihood choices they make.

Which factors affect transmission?

• Norms of entitlement determining access to capital • Economic trends and shocks • Access to and nature of markets • Presence, quality and accessibility of public, private and community-based social services and safety nets • HIV/AIDS pandemic; other regionally endemic diseases; stigma	• Structure of household and family • Child fostering practices • Education and skill level of parent(s) • Intent/attitude of parent(s) and child(ren) • Nature of living space

As indicated in table 3.1 and in box 3.1, below, intergenerational transfers are affected by the social, cultural, political, economic and institutional contexts in which they occur. While youth as a group face discrimination in many contexts, the extent to which poverty-related capital is transferred to a particular young person depends on the norms of entitlement associated with his or her gender, position among siblings and within the family, marital and parental status, and health status, as well as on behavioural factors such as parental and youth attitudes. Socially constructed norms of entitlement not only facilitate or constrain intergenerational transfers, but are often intergenerationally transferred themselves; discriminatory behaviour often endures across generations.

For both intergenerational poverty and life-course poverty,[10] processes are at work that may lead to or entrench poverty, as stylized in figure 3.3. Life-course poverty defines situations in which poor children or young people grow into poor, or even poorer, adults, while intergenerational poverty derives from transfers between individuals and households. Nonetheless, the processes occurring in connection with these two forms of poverty are often so closely related that distinctions can be difficult to make. For example, the inability of a parent to ensure that a child is provided with sufficient education may be said to reflect the intergenerational transmission of poverty, while an uneducated child growing into an unemployed adult may be interpreted as a consequence of life-course poverty. In practice, the processes work together.

Life-course poverty and intergenerational poverty can each be a cause, a characteristic, and an effect of chronic poverty. They constitute a cause in that certain types of deprivation, suffered to certain extents and experienced at particular points in the life course (especially, but not exclusively, during early childhood), can inflict damage that is difficult or even impossible to reverse later in life. They represent a characteristic in that the defining feature of chronic poverty is its persistence over time, so poverty that lasts throughout the life cycle and/or is passed on to the next generation is by definition chronic. Finally, they represent an effect based on evidence suggesting that the longer poverty lasts, the more difficult it becomes to escape. It is reported that in the United States of America, for example, people who have been in poverty for more than four years face a 90 per cent probability of remaining poor for the rest of their lives (Yaqub, 2000). If one or more of the assets (including income, social relationships and psychological resilience) of individuals or households fall below a "critical level",[11] it can become increasingly difficult for them to move from survival to improvement strategies.

It is important to disaggregate poverty figures by age in order to determine the extent to which an additional year of poverty during infancy, childhood or youth, for example, has a greater or lesser effect on one's ability to escape poverty than does an additional year of poverty in adulthood. The timing of poverty spells — even those that are relatively short — also matters, as does the timing of interventions (Yaqub, 2002). Figure 3.4 illustrates this assertion.

Figure 3.3
Stylization of intergenerationally transmitted and life-course poverty

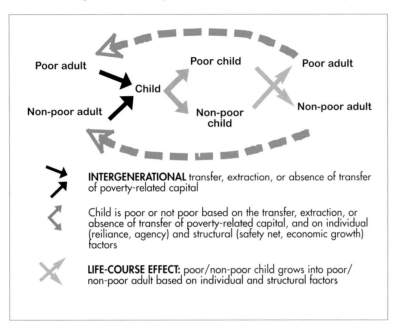

Source: "Frameworks for understanding the intergenerational transmission of poverty and well-being in developing countries", CPRC Working Paper No. 8 (Manchester, United Kingdom, Institute for Development Policy and Management/Chronic Poverty Research Centre, 2001).

Figure 3.4
Timing matters: an adaptation of Yaqub's "born poor, stay poor?" thesis

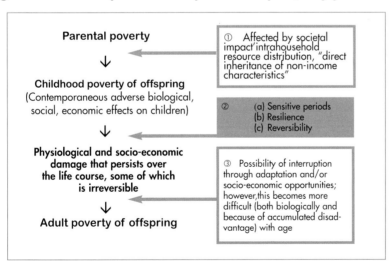

Source: Adapted from S. Yaqub, "Intertemporal welfare dynamics: extent and causes" (2000) (available from http://www.ceip.org/files/pdf/shahin_dynamics.pdf; accessed 1 October 2004); S. Yaqub, "At what age does poverty damage most? Exploring a hypothesis about 'timetabling' error in antipoverty", a paper presented at the Conference on Justice and Poverty: Examining Sen's Capability Approach, Cambridge, United Kingdom, 5-7 June 2001; and S. Yaqub, "Poor children grow into poor adults: harmful mechanisms or over-deterministic theory?", *Journal of International Development*, vol. 14, No. 8 (2002), pp. 1081-1093.

The distribution of resources and care

The extent to which parents transmit poverty to their children is influenced by the manner in which resources and care are distributed within the household and society (*see the section on factors affecting transmission in table 3.1 for further elaboration*). Parents' investments in their children—in terms of time and capital spent on education and training, health and nutrition, and general care—are strongly affected by available resources and localized norms of entitlement surrounding gender, age and birth order, among other factors.

A study of social mobility and adolescent schooling gaps[12] in Latin America illustrates this point. For most countries in the region there is a "reverse gender gap" in education; however, within individual households, gender as well as birth timing and birth order often make a difference (Andersen, 2001). Teenagers born to 30-year-old heads of household experience about a 7 per cent smaller schooling gap, on average, than those born to 20-year-old heads of household. At a time when they must make decisions about their children's education, young parents are likely to be earning a relatively low and erratic income, so they may elect to postpone, reduce or avoid the formal and transactional costs of schooling. Larger numbers of siblings increase the schooling gap for young people in a family, except in situations where there is an older sister, in which case resources seem to be diverted from her to her younger siblings. "Thus, in a hypothetical family who raised first a girl, then a boy, and then a girl, the oldest sister would have a 0.52 year (or 24 per cent) greater schooling gap than the younger sister. And this is not counting the life-cycle effect, which would further tend to increase the older sister's schooling gap compared to the younger sister's gap. The effects of siblings are larger in urban areas than rural areas." (Andersen, 2001, p. 30)

Box 3.1 provides an example of how some of these factors, including gendered norms of entitlement, family structure, parental education, and parental and child attitudes, interact to determine the level of investment in young people in the Philippines.

Inadequate education or training is often, though not always, a key factor constraining present and future livelihood opportunities. In a number of countries, the impact of women's education on the welfare of children (particularly that of girls in many cases) is much more significant than the impact of men's education. Demographic and Health Survey (DHS) data from the late 1990s suggest that in South-East Asia, where gender gaps in education are relatively low and education and literacy levels are relatively high (with the partial exceptions of Cambodia and the Lao People's Democratic Republic), economic and social factors limit the capacity of many young women to study beyond the primary level (ORC Macro, 2004). Overall, in the three countries for which relevant DHS data are available (Indonesia, the Philippines and Viet Nam), about 50 per cent of those women who left school at any time before completing higher education cited economic factors, and around 23 per cent cited marriage, pregnancy and/or childcare responsibilities, as the reasons for leaving. At the country level, just under two thirds of women in the Philippines cited economic factors, and more than 40 per cent of women in Indonesia cited marriage, as the reasons for discontinuing their education after completing secondary school.[13]

Box 3.1

HOW SOCIAL STRUCTURES AND PERCEPTIONS INFLUENCE
INVESTMENTS IN YOUNG PEOPLE IN RURAL AREAS OF THE PHILIPPINES

Two studies investigating the determinants of parental and/or grandparental investments in children in rural areas of the Philippines suggest that the factors affecting the intergenerational transmission of poverty-related capital can be highly contextual and complex.

The findings of one study[a] indicate that resource constraints, concerns about equity and efficiency, and risk-diversification strategies all play a part in decisions about investments in children and grandchildren, as detailed in the following:

- *The pre-marriage wealth of both parents and grandparents affects children's completed schooling levels.*

- *Grandparent wealth does not affect the distribution of education between grandsons and granddaughters, though it does affect the allocation of land.*

- *The influence of grandparents on children's schooling appears to work through physical proximity rather than through wealth.*

- *Sons are clearly favoured in terms of land inheritance, while daughters generally receive more education.*

- *Better-educated fathers favour daughters in terms of education, while mothers with more land favour sons.*

- *While there is no gender gap in education in the present-day Philippines, Filipino men continue to bring more land and other assets to marriage; this affects intrahousehold bargaining power and investments in the next generation.*

The other study[b] relates how parents' decisions about education depend on their perceptions of their children's inherent attitudes:

- *Parents in the Philippines invest in the schooling of girls because they are seen as "more studious", "patient", "willing to sacrifice", and "interested in their studies".*

- *Boys are seen as more prone to vices (such as drinking), are fond of "roaming around" and "playing with their barkada [peer group]", and have to be "reminded" and "scolded" to do their schoolwork.*

While not particularly straightforward, these types of findings can have important implications for a range of policy interventions in fields as diverse as education, property law, taxation and media.

---

[a] A. Quisumbing and K. Hallman, "Marriage in transition: evidence on age, education, and assets from six developing countries", Population Council/Policy Research Division, Working Paper No. 183 (December 2003).

[b] H.E. Bouis and others, "Gender equality and investments in adolescents in the rural Philippines", IFPRI Working Paper Series, Research Report No. 108 (Washington, D.C.: International Food Policy Research Institute, 1998).

The particulars relating to women's limited educational attainment in four East Asian countries are summarized in the following:

- In Viet Nam, almost 30 per cent of women aged 20-24 years had only a primary education. Needing to help the family was the main reason girls stopped attending school before completing the primary cycle, and getting married was the strongest reason for leaving after finishing primary school.

- In the Philippines, almost 20 per cent of women aged 20-24 years had only a primary education. The inability to pay for school was the most important reason girls and young women stopped studying both after completing primary school and after completing secondary school.

- In Indonesia, the inability to pay for school was the most important reason girls and young women withdrew from education after completing primary school, and getting married was the strongest factor after completing secondary school.

- In Cambodia (in 2000), almost 80 per cent of women aged 20-24 years had only a primary education. No DHS data are available on the reasons for their leaving school.

National economic change can also have a significant impact on the intergenerational transmission of poverty-related capital. Analysis has been undertaken to determine the extent to which the liberalization process in Viet Nam during the 1990s affected socioeconomic indicators of inequality, including disparities in child survival. The findings show that under-five mortality rates varied little for the different income quintiles in the early 1990s; however, by the late 1990s, the under-five mortality rate for the poorest quintile was more than twice that for the richest quintile. These changes have been traced to reductions among the poor (but not among the better-off) in the coverage of some health services and in women's educational attainment (Wagstaff and Nguyen, 2002).

Sensitivity to poverty

The extent to which the contemporaneous adverse biological, social and economic effects of parental poverty on a child lead to long-term functional physiological and socioeconomic damage depends on when the person experienced poverty, how resilient that person and his or her environment are to the effects of poverty, and the extent to which the damage inflicted is functionally reversible (*also see figure 3.4*).

Human beings are most sensitive to the negative effects of poverty, manifested in inadequate health and nutrition, in the womb and during the first few years of life (Yaqub, 2002). Growth and development, especially of the brain and immune system, during these sensitive foetal and early childhood periods can lay the groundwork for future cognitive and physical capacity, and possibly for more socioculturally dependent qualities such as behaviour. The long-term effects of poor nutrition in utero and in early childhood on physical and cognitive development are considered to be largely irreversible.

Children born to low-income adolescent girls are often especially susceptible to persistent poverty,[14] which may become more deeply entrenched over generations. Girls who grow up stunted or anaemic are more likely to be underdeveloped for childbirth and therefore face higher risks of maternal and child mortality, and of low birth weight and stunting among their own children (Commission on Nutrition Challenges of the 21st Century, 2000). These risks are often compounded by the earlier childbearing among poorer women in comparison with their better-off counterparts. As mentioned previously, an estimated 17 per cent of births in least developed countries are among women below the age of 20, which translates into 14 million births worldwide each year (United Nations Population Fund, 2004). The babies of these young women generally have a lower birth weight and are less healthy than the babies of older and better nourished women, and are thus more likely to suffer the harmful long-term (and often cyclical) effects described earlier. In most developing countries, teenage pregnancy is higher in rural areas and among women with no education or only a primary education.[15]

Certain factors, including personality traits (such as resilience) and different forms of support offered within the larger environment (such as schooling geared towards people with learning disabilities), can help young people overcome early disadvantages and prevent physiological damage from becoming a functional impairment.

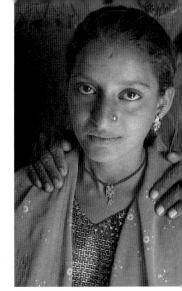

Foetal and childhood deprivation does not necessarily mean lifelong poverty, but interrupting life-course poverty requires adaptation as well as socio-economic opportunities. "Socio-economic attainments require a sound basis at each life stage" (Yaqub, 2002). However, avoiding or escaping poverty becomes more difficult with age, as both biological and socio-economic disadvantages accumulate. This highlights the central importance of adolescence and young adulthood—the period during which individuals begin to engage in most aspects of adult functioning, including sexual reproduction, labour market participation, and capital accumulation. In many contexts, after maternal and early childhood interventions are undertaken to prevent further harm, the provision of socio-economic opportunities and support for youth and young parents may be the most effective way to avert or interrupt intergenerational and life-course poverty. Actions that might be taken in this regard are outlined below in the section on policy implications.

CHILDHOOD DEPRIVATION AND ESTIMATES OF YOUTH POVERTY

In a recently released report financed by UNICEF, an innovative child-centred methodology has been used to measure the depth and extent of child poverty in developing regions (Gordon and others, 2003). An alternative measure of child poverty has been derived based on a set of indicators of severe deprivation of basic human needs, the argument being that it is not enough to base estimates of childhood poverty on household income, expenditure or consumption profiles alone, as poverty is also characterized by limited access to public goods such as safe drinking water and sanitation, roads, health care and education.

This approach is relevant to the discussion of youth poverty because (a) a proportion of those identified as "children" (individuals in the age group 15-18) may also be categorized as "youth"; (b) the remaining children will soon become youth; and (c) the authors have constructed their measure of childhood poverty to highlight aspects of deprivation that can be expected to have negative implications for well-being in both the short and long term.

The indicators of severe deprivation among children are as follows:

- *Severe food deprivation:* children whose height and weight for their age are more than three standard deviations below the median of the international reference population, signalling severe anthropometric failure (a failure to grow at a normal rate to a "normal" weight and height);

- *Severe water deprivation:* children who only have access to surface water (such as rivers) for drinking or who live in households where the nearest source of water is more than 15 minutes away (indicators of severe deprivation of water quality or quantity);

- *Severe deprivation of sanitation facilities:* children who have no access to sanitation facilities of any kind in the vicinity of their dwelling, that is, no private or communal toilets or latrines;

- *Severe health deprivation:* children who have not been immunized against any diseases or young children who have had a recent illness involving diarrhoea and did not receive any medical advice or treatment;

- *Severe shelter deprivation:* children in dwellings with more than five people per room (severe overcrowding) or with no flooring material (for example, a mud floor);

- *Severe educational deprivation:* children between the ages of 7 and 18 who have never been to school and are not currently attending school (no professional education of any kind);

- *Severe information deprivation:* children between the ages of 3 and 18 with no access to radio, television, telephone or newspapers at home;

- *Severe deprivation of access to basic services:* children living 20 kilometres (km) or more from any type of school or at least 50 km from any medical facility with doctors. (For the report financed by UNICEF, this information was available only for a few countries, so it was not possible to construct accurate regional estimates of severe deprivation of access to basic services.)

Survey data on nearly 1.2 million children in 46 countries, collected mainly during the late 1990s, were used for the UNICEF-sponsored report. The results of the analysis indicate that more than one half (over 1 billion) of the children in developing countries suffer from severe deprivation of at least one basic human need, and over one third (674 million) suffer from absolute poverty, signified by two or more severe deprivations. The highest rates of absolute poverty are found in sub-Saharan Africa (65 per cent, or 207 million children) and in South Asia (59 per cent, or 330 million children). The rates are lowest in Latin America and the Caribbean and in East Asia and the Pacific, at 17 and 7 per cent respectively. Rural children experience significantly higher levels of poverty than do urban children; rates of absolute poverty are 70 per cent or above in the rural areas of both South Asia and sub-Saharan Africa. Severe deprivation of shelter and sanitation facilities affects the highest proportion of children in the developing world-again, mainly in rural areas (Gordon and others, 2003).[16]

The report suggests that priority should be given to improving basic infrastructure and services for families with children, with particular attention focused on ensuring the availability of adequate shelter, sanitation and safe drinking water in rural areas. From a broader strategic perspective, it is emphasized that "in order to eradicate absolute poverty amongst children, policies will need to be targeted at the various problems they face. A single set of anti-poverty policies for the planet is not the most effective or efficient way to eradicate child poverty." (Gordon and others, 2003, p. 31)

These findings highlight the need for greater investment in efforts to achieve the child-focused Millennium Development Goals, as the young people of 2015 and beyond stand to benefit enormously. They also support the integration of policies for children and youth into national poverty reduction and overall development strategies-a step some countries have already taken.

Young people make up a significant proportion of the population in developing countries and, on grounds of equity alone, should constitute the focus for a significant proportion of national and global anti-poverty investments (Curtain, 2004). Moreover, in many contexts, youth may be disproportionately susceptible to poverty in comparison with other age groups, primarily owing to the extremely fluid nature of the challenges and opportunities they face during the transition to adulthood, particularly in relation to the labour market. This brief review of the interrelated concepts of chronic, life-course, intergenerational and youth poverty provides further justification for targeting youth in anti-poverty policies and programmes. Poverty experienced in youth not only has implications across the life course of a young person; it can also undermine that individual's capacity to bounce back from deprivation suffered in childhood and affect the long-term life chances of any dependants, especially the young person's own children.

The four-part action framework for confronting chronic poverty outlined in the *Chronic Poverty Report, 2004-05* is equally relevant to youth poverty (Chronic Poverty Research Centre, 2004, p. 50).

First is the need to prioritize livelihood security. Much greater emphasis should be placed on preventing and mitigating the shocks and insecurities that create and sustain chronic poverty. This involves not only providing recovery assistance but also giving chronically poor people a secure position from which to seize opportunities and demand their rights. For youth, for those on whom they depend, and for those who depend on them, three priorities must be set:

- Interrupt downward trajectories and allow opportunities to be pursued through the adoption of innovative social protection policies. Appropriate policy mechanisms and measures might include insurance systems and direct transfers, as well as non-contributory pensions (relevant for youth, who often have older dependants as well as their own future old age to consider). Youth-targeted social protection may include "hardship funds" that can be deployed to ensure that structural or atypical shocks do not push a young person out of secondary, tertiary or vocational education, or to support re-entry into the education system.

- Focus on preventing ill health and the descent into chronic poverty it can cause by, for example, providing preventive and curative services for breadwinners and caregivers. Universal free health care for mothers and young children can go a long way in protecting the lives and livelihoods of young people throughout the developing world.

- Focus on preventing and interrupting childhood poverty, primarily through interventions in nutrition, health, education and household security.

Second is the need to ensure that chronically poor people can take advantage of opportunities. It is argued that "pro-poor growth is the single most important measure for tackling youth unemployment" (Save the Children/Childhood Poverty Research and Policy Centre, 2004); however, growth of any kind (even pro-poor growth) is not enough to alleviate poverty in its most extreme and chronic forms. It is crucial both to promote broad-based growth and to facilitate the equitable redistribution of material and other assets so that chronically poor people can take up economic opportunities.

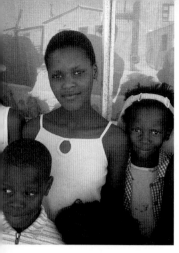

Making markets work for poor people, including making labour markets work for disadvantaged youth, is essential but difficult. In most contexts, efforts are needed to forge a closer link between educational provision and economic requirements. Priority should be given to increasing the quality and relevance of education and training, ensuring that young people stay in education long enough to develop the required skills, and combining training programmes with, for example, job search assistance, placement schemes, wage subsidies or access to credit, childcare or transportation (Save the Children/Childhood Poverty Research and Policy Centre, 2004).

Third is the need to take empowerment seriously. Policies must address the difficult political process of challenging the layers of discrimination that keep people trapped in poverty. For many youth, age-based discrimination adds to the discrimination they face because of their gender, ethnicity or poverty status. Young people can be effective agents of change within their communities. There is an urgent need to remove the political, legal and social barriers that work against vulnerable youth and other poor and chronically poor people in order to enhance their capacity to influence institutions that affect their lives.

Fourth is the need to recognize obligations to provide resources. Chronic poverty cannot be seriously reduced without real transfers of resources and sustained, predictable finance. Political indifference to fulfilling national and international poverty eradication commitments and obligations must be challenged and ways found to foster social solidarity across households, communities and countries. The need for policy change should not obscure the fact that it is the chronically poor themselves that are working hardest to overcome their poverty. Even now, when their existence is recognized, the chronically poor—and particularly poor children, youth, older people and persons with disabilities—are perceived in both policy circles and the popular imagination as dependent and passive. Nothing could be further from the truth. Most people in chronic poverty are striving to improve their livelihoods and prospects for their families under difficult circumstances not of their own choosing. They need real commitment at the highest levels, backed up by action and resources, to support their efforts to secure their rights and overcome the obstacles that trap them in poverty.

CONCLUSION

Youth poverty is a serious development problem, not least because of the large numbers of young people living in absolute poverty in developing countries; as indicated in the present and preceding chapters, this group includes about 674 million individuals under the age of 18 and around 209 million between the ages of 15 and 24. In many contexts, youth are more likely to experience poverty than those in other age groups because of the uncertainties and dynamism characterizing the transition from childhood to adulthood (particularly with regard to relationships and responsibilities), or owing to age-based discrimination, especially in labour markets.

As elaborated in this chapter, however, context matters, and the relative extent of youth poverty in a given community or country depends on the interaction of many different factors. In settings in which young people—or particular groups of youth such as young women, indigenous youth, or youth with disabilities—are disproportionately poor or vulnerable to poverty, understanding what has driven and maintained this poverty is crucial for developing effective policy interventions. Falling into, becoming stuck in, or escaping from poverty during youth (or at any other stage of the life cycle) is based on variable combinations of structural and idiosyncratic factors and life-course events occurring in a multitude of contexts ranging from the individual to the global. After early childhood, adolescence and young adulthood may be the period in which anti-poverty interventions have the greatest potential to effect long-term positive change.

The related concepts of chronic poverty, life-course poverty and intergenerational poverty contribute to a better understanding of youth poverty. First, an analysis of the multiple and interacting causes of chronic poverty can help identify the relative positions of different groups of poor people, facilitating policy prioritization in contexts of resource scarcity. Second, life-course events and experiences such as leaving school, starting work, getting married and having children can seriously affect a person's vulnerability to poverty. These and other critical events are likely to occur at particular stages of the life cycle; as previously mentioned, these stages are not necessarily defined by age and are highly contextual. Third, it is important to adopt an intergenerational perspective because poverty experienced in youth is often linked to parental poverty (manifested in poor maternal nutrition or inadequate shelter, for example) and childhood deprivation (such as being forced to leave school early or engage in dangerous work); in addition, youth poverty—like poverty experienced in childhood or old age—can have implications across the life course of a young person and that of his or her household.

Qualitative and quantitative cross-sectional research has provided a deeper understanding of the dynamics of poverty during youth and other stages of the life course. The processes driving or maintaining poverty change over time, often very rapidly in the context of large-scale political or economic shocks. Ongoing construction and analysis of qualitative and quantitative panel data sets with information on poverty over the life course and across generations, particularly for developing countries, can provide an effective means of indicating to policymakers the types and timings of anti-poverty interventions required. ●

---

[1] For the sake of simplicity, the word "parents" in this chapter is used to signify older generations of individuals responsible for the well-being of children. The often significant role of grandparents, siblings and other relatives and non-relatives is duly acknowledged.

[2] This child-centred approach to estimating childhood deprivation has been described in *Child Poverty in the Developing World* (Gordon and others, 2003).

[3] In the *Chronic Poverty Report, 2004-05*, this is illustrated by the story of Maymana and Mofizul, who make up a household in rural Bangladesh; their chronic poverty is an outcome of ill-health, widowhood, a saturated rural labour market, disability, social injustice and poor governance, among other factors (Chronic Poverty Research Centre, 2004).

[4] Adapted from the Chronic Poverty Report, 2004-05 (Chronic Poverty Research Centre, 2004).

[5] For a discussion of how a stagnant economy along with widespread social exclusion of a large and educated youth population laid the groundwork for the emergence and maintenance of political conflict in Sri Lanka; see the "Economic roots of political conflict: the case of Sri Lanka" (Abeyratne, 2004).

[6] The ratio of economically active household members to those who are economically dependent. Children, older people, the ill and the disabled are generally considered dependants, although each may contribute directly or indirectly to household income and consumption.

[7] In contrast, the United States Panel Study of Income Dynamics (PSID) (http://psidonline.isr.umich.edu/) has collected data annually since 1968. By 2001, the original 4,800 households had grown to over 7,000. At the conclusion of the 2003 wave of data collection, the PSID will have collected information about more than 65,000 individuals spanning a period of up to 36 years of their lives. The British Household Panel Survey (http://iserwww.essex.ac.uk/ulsc/bhps/) has collected annual data over 13 years on 5,500 sample households, new members in those households, and "spin-off" households when individuals have left. Both panels are regularly supplemented with other large samples on topics of interest, such as child development.

[8] For further discussion of issues surrounding poverty-related longitudinal research, see "Urban Longitudinal Research Methodology: background paper written for the joint DPU-ODI-DFID-World Bank Workshop" (Moser, 2003).

[9] In chapter 2 of this publication, Curtain states that "existing research may be overly focused on groups living in chronic poverty". This is not strictly true. "Static" (cross-sectional) surveys measure whoever is poor at a particular moment, so both the temporarily and the chronically poor are measured, but there is no way of distinguishing between the two.

Consider a population with 10 households, two of which are "never poor", and two of which are "always poor". The remaining 60 per cent are transitorily poor; some fall into poverty every few years owing to an economic or climatic shock, while others face a lean season every year. The extent to which these households are captured by a cross-sectional survey completely depends on which year, season or month the survey is undertaken.

Curtain's point that "young people in poverty are likely to be underrepresented in (household surveys) if they have left the parental home and are in precarious circumstances, perhaps living in temporary accommodations or in no accommodations at all" is well-taken. This is not, however, an argument in favour of either cross-sectional or panel surveys, but an argument to do all surveys differently.

Further, in any given country, both the extent to which youth (defined as those aged 15-24 years) live in such situations, and the relative extent to which young people are disproportionately represented (compared with other mobile groups including migrant labourers), remain empirical questions.

[10] Life-course poverty is also sometimes referred to as intragenerational poverty, though this can also mean poverty-related transfers within a generational cohort (that is, between same-generation peers or family members).

[11] Other authors have referred to this "critical level" as "ratchets" (Chambers, 1983) and as "accumulated disadvantage" (Yaqub, 2001).

[12] An "adolescent schooling gap" is defined by L.E. Andersen (2001, p. 8) as the "disparity between the years of education that a teenager or young adult would have completed had she entered school at normal school starting age and advanced one grade each year, on one hand, and the actual years of education, on the other hand. Thus, the schooling gap measures years of missing education." Teenagers are here defined as those aged 13-19 years; only "those still living at home" are included in the analysis. The "reverse gender gap" in education describes the situation in most Latin American countries, where female teenagers have more education than their male counterparts. In the developing world as a whole, the situation is reversed. Andersen's analysis suggests that the overall reverse gender gap in education does not, however, appear to lead to the expected higher social mobility among female teenagers in comparison with male teenagers.

[13] In other countries for which there are relatively recent data on women who left school at any time before completing higher education, the proportions who cited economic factors as the reason for leaving ranged from only 7 per cent in Jordan (1997) and Turkey (1998) to 47 per cent in Bolivia (1998). Over one half of Bolivian and Nepali women cited economic factors as the reason for leaving before completing primary school. The proportions of women who cited marriage or children as the reason for leaving school ranged from only 5 per cent in Turkey to 58 per cent in Jordan. Over three quarters of Nepali and Jordanian women cited marriage or children as factors in their leaving after completing secondary school or, for Nepali women, before completing higher education.

[14] Also see Buvinic (1998).

[15] These differences are often extreme. For example, in Benin in 2001, teenage pregnancy was 2.5 times higher in rural than in urban areas, over twice as common among those with no education compared with those that had a primary education, and over 6.5 times as common among those with no education compared with those that had a secondary education or higher.

[16] Severe deprivation is defined as "those circumstances that are highly likely to have serious adverse consequences for the health, well-being and development of children. Severe deprivations are causally related to 'poor' developmental outcomes both long and short term" (Gordon and others, 2003). Indicators have been developed for severe deprivation based on the absence of food, water, sanitation facilities, health, shelter, education, information and access to basic services. A child is living in absolute poverty only if he or she suffers from two or more severe deprivations of basic human needs.

Bibliography

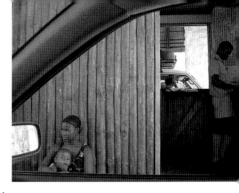

Abeyratne, S. (2004). Economic roots of political conflict: the case of Sri Lanka. *The World Economy*, vol. 7, No. 28 (August), pp. 1295-1314.

Andersen, L.E. (2001). Social mobility in Latin America: links with adolescent schooling. IADB Research Network Working Paper No. R-433. Washington, D.C.: Inter-American Development Bank, July.

Buvinic, M. (1998). Costs of adolescent childbearing: a review of evidence from Chile, Barbados, Guatemala and Mexico. IADB Sustainable Development Department Paper No. WID-102. Washington, D.C.: Inter-American Development Bank, July.

Chambers, R. (1983). *Rural Development—Putting the Last First*. Harlow, Essex, United Kingdom: Longman Scientific & Technical.

Chronic Poverty Research Centre (2004). *Chronic Poverty Report, 2004-05*. Manchester, United Kingdom: Institute for Development Policy and Management/CPRC.

Commission on the Nutrition Challenges of the 21st Century (2000). Ending malnutrition by 2020: an agenda for change in the millennium. *Food and Nutrition Bulletin*, vol. 21, No. 3, supplement (September). Tokyo: United Nations University Press.

Curtain, R. (2004). Youth in extreme poverty: dimensions and country responses. *World Youth Report, 2003: The Global Situation of Young People*. United Nations publication, Sales No. E.03.IV.7.

Gordon, D., and others (2003). *Child Poverty in the Developing World*. Bristol: The Policy Press.

International Labour Organization (2004). Global Employment Trends for Youth. Geneva.

Moser, C., ed. (2003). Urban Longitudinal Research Methodology: background paper written for the joint DPU-ODI-DFID-World Bank Workshop, May 28th—29th 2003. DPU Working Paper No. 124.

ORC Macro (2004). Measure DHS STATcompiler (available from http://www.measuredhs.com).

Rigg, J., and T. Sefton (2004). Income dynamics and the life cycle. Centre for Analysis of Social Exclusion Paper No. 81. London: London School of Economics.

Save the Children/Childhood Poverty Research and Policy Centre (2004). Promoting disadvantaged young people's employment: What can be done? CHIP Briefing 61. London.

United Kingdom, British Household Panel Survey (available from http://iserwww.essex.ac.uk/ulsc/bhps/).

United Nations Population Fund (2004). *State of the World's Population, 2004—The Cairo Consensus at Ten: Population, Reproductive Health and the Global Effort to End Poverty*. New York.

_____ (2005). *Young People as part of a National Poverty Reduction Strategy: Reference Notes on Population and Poverty Reduction*. New York.

United States, Panel Study of Income Dynamics (available from http://psidonline.isr.umich.edu/)

Wagstaff, A., and N.N. Nguyen (2002). Poverty and survival prospects of Vietnamese children under Doi Moi. World Bank Policy Research Working Paper No. 2832. Washington, D.C.: World Bank.

Yaqub, S. (2000). Intertemporal welfare dynamics: extent and causes. Brighton, United Kingdom: Poverty Research Unit AFRAS, Sussex University (available from http://www.ceip.org/files/pdf/shahin_dynamics.pdf; accessed 1 October 2004).

_____ (2001). At what age does poverty damage most? Exploring a hypothesis about "timetabling" error in antipoverty. Paper presented to the Conference on Justice and Poverty: Examining Sen's Capability Approach, Cambridge, United Kingdom, 5-7 June. Cambridge: 21 May.

_____ (2002). Poor children grow into poor adults: harmful mechanisms or over-deterministic theory?" *Journal of International Development*, vol. 14, No. 8, pp. 1081-1093.

YOUTH in

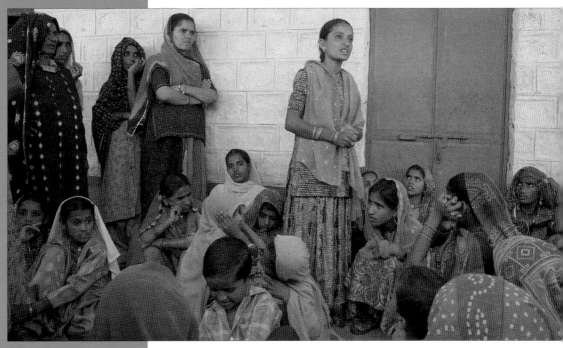

Civil
Society

PART TWO

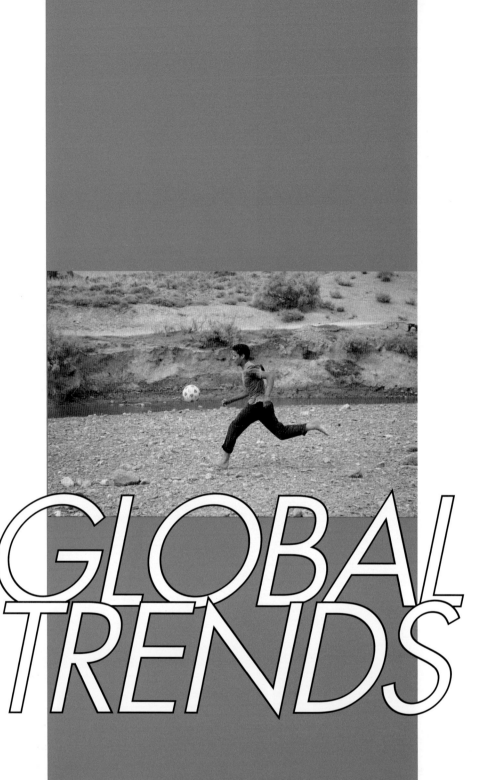

GLOBAL TRENDS

Chapter 4

By virtue of their membership in a family unit, a neighbourhood, a school district, a cultural group, and a multitude of other community building blocks, young people both shape and are shaped by the society around them. This second part of the publication examines the priority issues for youth development that relate to the dynamics between young people and their societies. It begins by outlining how young people view the environment, highlighting their role as the vanguard in sustainable development and its application to their local surroundings. Another focus is leisure-time activities and the growing awareness of the vital contribution discretionary hours make to the social inclusion of young people in their societies. Participation in decision-making is the third major area explored, in recognition of the fact that young people need to be involved in the processes that help shape their socio-economic environment.

Within the context of the five new areas of concern recognized by the United Nations since the adoption of the World Programme of Action for Youth to the Year 2000 and Beyond, this part also examines two important developments that have brought about significant changes in the socialization and participation of young people. One is the ageing of societies, which has profound implications for intergenerational relations. The other is the expansion of information and communication technology (ICT), the multiple dimensions of which were still emerging when the Programme of Action for Youth was adopted in 1995.

When considered in connection with priorities such as leisure-time activities or participation in decision-making, it becomes apparent that ICT has contributed enormously to the development of a global media-driven youth culture. The effects of this emerging culture are increasingly identifiable in the lives of many young people and are altering socialization patterns, processes and experiences. The magnitude and implications of this trend make it imperative that a closer look be taken at what it means to grow up in a global media-driven youth culture. Chapters 5 and 6 of this part of the publication focus specifically on how this dynamic is creating new forms of socialization within societies, the implications of new media for young people, and the influence of these media on young people's participation and civic engagement.

ENVIRONMENT

Recognizing that they will bear the consequences of current environmental policies, young people continue to have a strong interest in protecting and preserving the planet's resources. The participation of young people in the United Nations Conference on Environment and Development in 1992 set the stage for participation by youth groups in other global conferences, culminating in their relatively high-profile involvement in the World Summit on Sustainable Development, held in Johannesburg in 2002.

The environment-related proposals in the World Programme of Action for Youth are reinforced in the Johannesburg Plan of Implementation. The World Programme of Action calls for mainstreaming environmental education and training in general school curricula and training programmes. Throughout the process surrounding the World Summit on Sustainable Development, young people advocated for renewed commitment to education for sustainable development. At its fifty-seventh session in December 2002, the General Assembly proclaimed 2005-2014 the United Nations Decade of Education for Sustainable Development. The International Implementation Scheme for the Decade establishes a broad framework for all partners, including youth, to contribute to its activities.

Environmental education has grown steadily over the past decade through its inclusion in both school curricula and non-formal and informal educational programmes. Increasing numbers of national and regional professional associations of environmental educators are lending strength to this trend. However, the real challenge lies in achieving visible gains from environmental education, or in other words, translating environmental values into changes in behaviour, which requires increased political commitment and lifestyle adjustments. Environmental education should incorporate provisions for effecting well-designed and concrete changes. Working with young people at the local, grass-roots level to preserve the environment is critical to achieving the Millennium Development Goal of ensuring environmental sustainability.

The World Programme of Action for Youth proposes strengthening the participation of young people in the protection, preservation and improvement of the environment. Youth have been and continue to be actively involved in implementing environmental projects and in identifying new strategies for addressing environmental problems. Such experience qualifies them for increased participation in decisions relating to environmental policy. At a practical level, enhancing the role of young people in environmental protection will require their integration into the decision-making structures of government-supported programmes and non-governmental organizations.

Lessons can be drawn from the Tunza Youth Strategy adopted by the United Nations Environment Programme (UNEP) in 2003, which is designed to engage young people in the work of the organization and in a broad range of activities aimed at enhancing environmental conservation and sustainable development. At the annual Tunza International Youth Conference, young people take stock of the progress achieved with regard to the Johannesburg Plan of Implementation and review their role in promoting sustainable development within the UNEP framework.

The World Programme of Action for Youth recognizes the essential role of the media in the widespread dissemination of environmental information among young people. It is felt by many youth, however, that the mainstream media have not provided comprehensive reporting of environmental issues, so they are increasingly disseminating environmental information through their own channels. At the World Summit on Sustainable Development, the Global Youth Reporters Programme provided live news feeds offering a unique perspective on what world leaders were undertaking in the Johannesburg Plan of Implementation. Young people, who tend to adopt technology very rapidly, are increasingly using media such as camcorders, digital film editing software and the Internet to produce and distribute their own environmental material. Growing numbers of young people are relying on environmental films, videos, blogs (web logs featuring short Internet chats and journals), and zines (small handmade publications) to reach out to each other and share their environmental values and concerns.

The past decade has seen a shift in perceptions regarding the role of leisure-time activities in a young person's development. In the traditional view, leisure time is simply seen as "free time", but there has been a growing awareness of the vital contribution discretionary time can make to a young person's social inclusion, access to opportunities and overall development. Terms such as "leisure", "informal activities" and "free time" imply a casualness of purpose and practice that does not do justice to the way a majority of young people use their unrestricted hours. In many cases, young people's leisure time and activities relate directly to important issues affecting them, including education and employment. Out of both necessity and interest, they are increasingly seeking and finding new ways to spend their free time.

HIV/AIDS, delinquency, conflict, drug abuse and other threats to a young person's well-being constitute a particular danger during discretionary time; however, many projects and programmes designed to engage young people in more positive pursuits are focused on these very issues as well, though they may or may not be available in certain settings. Given such interconnections, it is critical that leisure-time activities be viewed within the overall context of youth development and the participation of young people in their communities and society.

In many industrialized countries, cuts in government subsidies for sports activities, music and art instruction, and other leisure and recreational options have endangered many valuable extracurricular programmes in and out of schools. The loss of these opportunities is producing greater numbers of latchkey children, who either return home to empty dwellings or roam the streets. Some young people are initiating projects in areas in which public programmes fall short, but they require assistance and support, including supervision, the provision of meeting places, and increased access to other public facilities. The leisure needs of young people must be considered in the processes of urban planning and rural development in order to ensure that they have access to a range of constructive voluntary activities and opportunities.

Leisure activities in which young people are positively engaged in volunteerism are particularly important, as statistics show that individuals who volunteer in their youth are more likely to continue to do so in their later years. Some studies in North America show that young volunteers are more likely to do well in school and to vote. The International Year of Volunteers in 2001 played an important part in broadening traditional perceptions of the nature, role and contributions of young people as volunteers. By the end of that year, there was a general consensus in the international community that the canvas of youth volunteerism encompassed, but was much broader than, leisure-time activities. Young people volunteer in a number of ways, engaging in activism, participating in formal service organizations, and even assuming responsibilities within mutual aid systems, which are particularly prevalent in developing countries. The momentum generated during the International Year of Volunteers must be sustained, as volunteerism has the potential to engage large numbers of young people in activities that can contribute greatly to the achievement of the Millennium Development Goals.

There has been increasing affirmation of the connection between leisure-time sports activities and development, as participation in sports not only improves physical health, but also contributes to the development of a positive self-concept and essential social skills and values such as teamwork and tolerance. Furthermore, sport is a universal language that brings all types of people together, regardless of their origin, background, religious beliefs or economic status. It cuts across barriers that divide societies, making it a powerful tool for promoting positive goals such as conflict prevention and peace-building among young people, both symbolically at the global level and more practically within communities. Well-designed sport-based initiatives are practical, cost-effective mechanisms for achieving peace and development objectives.

An increasing number of variables are determining how young people make use of their time outside of school or work. Universally high levels of youth unemployment and the rising costs associated with higher education often compel young people to limit their leisure pursuits to career exploration and preparation activities that facilitate the transition from school to work. This trend helps explain the sustained decline in memberships in sports associations and other organized forms of leisure activity.

ICT has also affected leisure-time habits, as social interaction is increasingly taking place within an electronic environment through such means as text messaging and online meetings. New leisurely pursuits such as downloading music, using instant messages, and playing electronic games are for the most part solitary activities. Some of these pastimes are replacing more traditional pursuits, such as sports. A Norwegian study indicates that children and young people are spending less time participating in physical recreation and sporting activities, and that only 47 per cent of young people between the ages of 20 and 24 engage in physical training of any kind every 14 days (or more often) (Mjaavatn, 1999). The development of modern technologies may be contributing to the evolution of a culture of "individualized leisure" as young people increasingly devote their free time to computer screens and mobile keypads.

PARTICIPATION IN DECISION-MAKING

The past decade has seen a growing acceptance of the importance of youth participation in decision-making, and successful efforts to engage young people in the political process have led to improved policy formulation, adoption, implementation and evaluation. Participation strengthens young people's commitment to and understanding of the concepts of human rights and democracy. The traditional view that "youth are the future" fails to take into account that young people are very active contributors to their societies today.

While involving young people in the decisions that affect society is beneficial from both a policymaking and a youth development perspective, it is not always effectively practised. The nature of youth engagement ranges from manipulation and tokenism to the assumption of full responsibility for the design and implementation of programmatic responses. Effective youth participation requires fundamental changes in the way societies perceive young people. To induce such changes it is necessary to provide adequate funding, introduce innovative ways to spread information, furnish training to facilitate intergenerational collaboration, and create organizational structures that welcome new voices. Strategies for youth participation must move away from ad hoc, activity-based

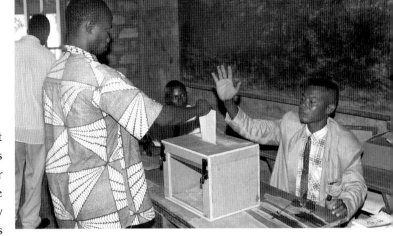

approaches and focus instead on making youth input a central component of social structures, institutions and processes. Efforts should be undertaken to foster intergenerational relationships and strengthen the capacity of young people to participate meaningfully and equally with other generations in programmes and activities that affect them. Girls and young women, in particular, may need additional support to overcome social, cultural, and economic barriers to full participation.

In national efforts to include youth in decision-making, consideration must be given to the changes occurring in the political attitudes of young people and in the patterns and structures of youth movements. In many countries, political parties are having difficulty attracting young members. Campaigns that encourage youth to vote seek to reverse the trend of reduced political interest among young people. Apathy towards politics and a lack of interest in joining traditional youth organizations seem to characterize the younger generation in many countries. To many young people, the world of politics seems far removed from their daily realities of school commitments, leisure activities, and employment challenges. Many youth fail to see a connection between these realities and the impact of public policies on their lives. Low voter turnout and dwindling membership in political parties should not lead to the conclusion that young people are uninterested in the political future of their societies. Although most student movements are still confined to university settings, the range of student-driven causes has expanded beyond educational reform and funding cuts to include democratic reforms, employment and health issues, racism, arms proliferation, environmental challenges, and a host of other concerns. Student movements have played a crucial role in a number of major social and political transitions that have occurred in various countries in recent history and are likely to continue to be at the forefront of the struggle for democratization and progressive social action.

In many countries, local, regional and national youth councils are major outlets for political and civic participation. Youth councils and forums, which may vary in terms of structure and mandate, have been the traditional channels through which young people have cooperated and communicated with national authorities and other decision makers. In a number of settings, however, these youth structures face an uncertain future, as the stable public funding they need to remain viable can no longer be guaranteed and is often not available in developing or transition countries. Many youth organizations must be results-focused and project-driven in order to receive funding. An interesting irony is that because formal youth councils are often mirrors of the political structures currently in place, some young people feel they are being asked to participate in the very same structures that they believe preclude true and effective participation. Some studies indicate that the motivation for joining formal youth organizations is changing, with many members having a pragmatic rather than an ideological interest in their activities. Membership is increasingly viewed as a way to enhance a young person's career or other prospects rather than as an opportunity to advance youth-driven ideas and policies.

While the importance of participation and its role in a young person's life has not diminished, its nature has changed. Youth participation today tends to be issue-specific and service-oriented. Increasingly reluctant to join formal organizations or councils, many young people prefer to take advantage of open opportunities created by communities and institutions to become involved in addressing the issues that concern them. In line with this trend, new participatory structures have evolved that tend to be based on collaborative networks and common interests. One popular option that seems to be playing an important role in reversing the decline in traditional participation and civic engagement among youth is Internet-based activity involving the exchange of ideas and information and the coordination of plans and programmes for localized action. Through cross-boundary websites, tele- and video-conferencing, chat boards and webcams, ICT has facilitated the development of new forms of creative, open and non-hierarchical channels of cyber-participation. Youth are gradually becoming more aware of resources outside their communities and of opportunities to share in and reinforce each other's work. While these new modes of participation are not substitutes for strong and effective youth councils, they can provide more young people with opportunities to become active in decision-making and in shaping their societies.

Policymakers should familiarize themselves with these new configurations and the types of activities in which young people are engaged in order to gain some insight into their concerns and priorities, and to provide whatever support is necessary to ensure that effective use is made of these new participatory opportunities. To ensure that effective participation is an option for all young people, explicit efforts must be made to address obstacles such as cultural norms that favour hierarchical relationships, economic circumstances that preclude participation in anything other than income-generating activities, and the lack of access to the information and skills necessary for active political involvement.

INTERGENERATIONAL RELATIONS

Before the middle of this century, older persons and children will comprise a roughly equal share of the world's population. The proportion of those aged 60 years and over is expected to double, rising from 10 to 21 per cent between 2000 and 2050, and the proportion of those under 14 years of age will decline by a third, from 30 to 20 per cent (*see figure 4.1*) (United Nations, 2003a). The youth population will decrease from 18 to 14 per cent of the total (United Nations, 2003c).

Figure 4.1
The global population, by age group, 2000, 2025 and 2050 (*Millions*)

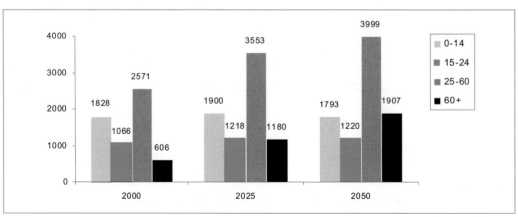

Source: United Nations, *World Population Prospects: The 2002 Revision; Volume II: Sex and Age* (Sales No. 03.XIII.7).

The ageing of society is already apparent in developed countries; however, the process is actually occurring much more rapidly in developing countries, and in many cases the necessary infrastructure and policies will not be in place to deal with the consequent developments. Today, 6 of every 10 older persons live in developing countries, but by 2050 the proportion is expected to rise to 8 in 10 (*see figure 4.2*). Africa remains the region with the youngest population; over time, however, the proportion of youth is expected to decline and the proportion of older persons will likely double.

Figure 4.2
The proportions of youth and older persons in the total
world population, 2000 and 2050

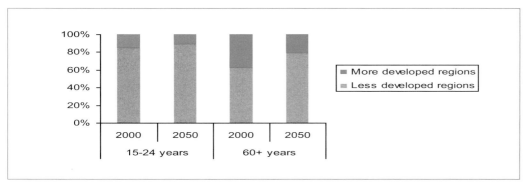

Source: United Nations, *World Population Prospects: The 2002 Revision;
Volume II: Sex and Age* (Sales No. 03.XIII.7).

Between 2000 and 2050, average life expectancy is expected to increase from 65 to 74 years (United Nations, 2003b). Consequently, families consisting of four or more generations will not be uncommon. This raises questions about the responsibilities of individuals within the family and the capacities of welfare systems to meet old-age pension and health-care needs. The interdependence between younger and older people will increase in the future. Youth development will become a more urgent prerequisite for meeting the growing care demands of older people and a condition for the development of society as a whole.

Related members of different generations continue to live with one another in the family context. However, family structures are undergoing profound changes. There has been a shift from extended to nuclear families and an increase in one-person households. The age at first marriage has risen to the mid- to late twenties in many areas, often owing to extended educational careers and delayed entry into the labour market, particularly for young women. There is also a trend towards later childbearing and having fewer children.

The AIDS pandemic has reversed decades of gradual gains in life expectancy in sub-Saharan Africa. In the worst-affected countries of eastern and southern Africa, the probability of a 15-year old dying before age 60 rose from between 10 and 30 per cent in the mid-1980s to between 30 and 60 per cent at the start of the new millennium (World Health Organization, 2004). The intergenerational impact of the epidemic has been felt most acutely by young people. Youth are frequently forced to take on new roles and responsibilities in their families and societies, caring for infected relatives, coping with the loss of family members, and raising their younger siblings orphaned by AIDS.

The extent to which a young person is economically dependent, independent or depended upon within the household can change extremely rapidly. This has important implications for the present and long-term well-being of both the young person and his or her family. Unemployment, which is relatively high among youth, prevents many young people from becoming economically independent from their families, or from contributing substantially to family well-being.

Intergenerational relations are also linked to cultural trends. In the transitional phase from childhood to adulthood, young people establish their own identities, adopting the cultural norms and values of their parents and adapting them to their own social and cultural environments. The globalization of media has expanded the scope of norms and values upon which young people draw in creating their identities. Young people are increasingly incorporating aspects of other cultures from around the world into their own identities. This trend, along with the "intergenerational digital divide", is likely to widen the cultural gaps between the younger and older generations.

Increased attention should be given to the socio-economic impact of ageing societies. A two-pronged approach may be adopted to address this issue at the most fundamental level: first, human development efforts should focus on different stages of the life course through age-adjusted policies and programmes that encourage workplace flexibility, lifelong learning and healthy lifestyles, with particular attention given to transitional periods such as youth to adulthood, family formation, and middle age to later years; and second, steps should be taken to strengthen the social environment at the family, neighbourhood and community levels.

INFORMATION AND
COMMUNICATION TECHNOLOGY

Young people are at the forefront of the technology revolution, which is the driving force behind the global emergence and evolution of the information- and knowledge-based society. Youth are often the leading innovators in the development, use and spread of ICT. They adapt quickly and are generally very eager to access the great quantities of local and global information made available through technological innovation.

A national survey conducted in the United States indicates that 91 per cent of young people aged 18-19 years use the Internet to e-mail friends and relatives, and 83 per cent use it for instant messaging. A recent study in the United Kingdom reveals that 94 per cent of youth have cell phones, and that young people were responsible for half of the roughly 10 billion text messages sent in 2003 (British Broadcasting Corporation, no date). Cell phone users are getting younger, and teenagers are spending more money on mobile communication every year. In 2001, the total number of mobile phone subscribers in the world stood at 860 million (Curtain, 2003). An average of 80 per cent of young people in the European Union use a mobile phone at least once a week (European Commission, no date). In China, nearly 60 per cent of cell phone subscribers are between 20 and 30 years of age.

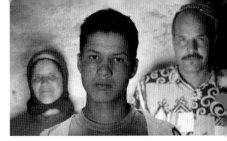

ICT has become a significant factor in development and is having a profound impact on the political, economic and social sectors in many countries. While many associate ICT primarily with mobile and more advanced technologies, a more useful definition of the term is one encompassing all technologies that enable the handling of information and facilitate different forms of communication. Expanding the characterization of ICT to include both older and newer technologies ranging from newspapers, radio and television to camcorders, computers and cell phones makes it possible to acquire a better understanding of the full impact of ICT on the social development of youth. The distinctions between old and new technologies may soon disappear as radio, television, satellite technologies and the Internet are combined in innovative ways to reach a wide range of target audiences.

The proliferation of ICT presents both opportunities and challenges with regard to the social development and inclusion of youth. Young people often use the Internet to access entertainment, news sites and virtual meeting spaces. They also utilize new technologies to participate in a number of civic activities. ICT is increasingly being used to improve access to education and employment opportunities, which supports efforts to eradicate poverty. However, while ICT clearly has the potential to empower young people and improve their lives in many respects, questions remain regarding its role in deepening existing inequalities and divisions in the world. The important concerns surrounding the global digital divide apply as much to youth as to any other age group.

There are still wide disparities in the distribution and utilization of many forms of technology. For example, 331 out of every 1,000 people in Europe use the Internet, but the same is true for only around 92 per 1,000 in Latin America and the Caribbean, 37 per 1,000 in the Middle East and North Africa, and 15 per 1,000 in South Asia and sub-Saharan Africa. Although these data are not age-specific, young people are among the principal users of computers and are likely highly represented in these figures. It is important to note that the disparities are not as great for the use of older forms of technology such as radio and television, which makes these media extremely useful for information distribution. For example, rates of radio ownership are 813 per 1,000 in Europe, 410 per 1,000 in Latin America and the Caribbean, 277 per 1,000 in the Middle East and North Africa, and 198 per 1,000 in sub-Saharan Africa (World Bank, 2004).

ICT access remains a major challenge for many young people. Rapid advances in wireless technology have made it possible to overcome the physical impediments of distance and topography that have limited the development of traditional telecommunications infrastructure in rural and other outlying areas; in other words, it is now theoretically possible to provide ICT services almost anywhere in the world at a relatively reasonable cost. Nonetheless, many poor youth are unable to take advantage of new technologies because of access limitations or cost factors. In the most remote and sparsely populated areas, there may not be enough of a market incentive for private investment in communications technologies, and government funding may be required. The digital divide, characterized by highly unequal ICT access and use, persists both within and between countries and should therefore be addressed by both national policymakers and the international community.

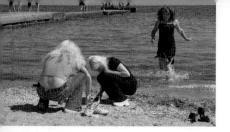

The terms cyber-participation and e-citizenship are indicative of a growing trend towards ICT-based social action and community development among young people. ICT and new media are becoming core components of youth activism and civic engagement. Because new technologies provide immediate and direct access to global information, young people have become more aware of issues, problems and crises in other parts of the world. These technologies are used by youth movements for communication and coordination, allowing instantaneous contact between young activists, and also serve to strengthen the sense of e-solidarity among individuals and groups with different agendas. In many countries, the Internet is the least-controlled information medium and can be a powerful tool for activists and advocacy groups, contributing to increased transparency, the development of civil society, and democracy. List servers, temporary and long-term websites, and collective online document writing and editing are common features of today's youth activism; these and other tools are commonly used by young people to prepare and contribute their submissions to international meetings and to facilitate their participation in political processes. This subject will be examined in greater depth in the coming chapters on the emergence of a global media-driven youth culture. Measures to improve Internet access and increase ICT literacy across the board will promote youth participation, and the effective use of technology should help to strengthen various forms of youth engagement.

ICT has the potential to improve young people's access to educational opportunities and to enhance the quality of education through new modes of learning. Many schools and vocational training centres are taking advantage of new technologies to provide distance learning and to train educators in new instructional methods. Digital opportunities are particularly beneficial for rural communities that lack libraries and other educational resources. Through ICT, curricula can be updated, adapted and even personalized to satisfy a broad range of learning needs, and can be distributed more effectively over a wider area. Even within the more traditional learning environments, technology is changing the way classrooms operate; the integration of multimedia subject presentation, online research, changing teacher-student dynamics, and innovative project approaches are making the learning process more interactive and participatory. ICT is only useful in improving educational access and quality if it is widely accessible and used appropriately; fortunately, cost-effective and country-differentiated solutions have been developed that may be used or adapted to address these issues.

ICT has been increasingly used to promote youth employment over the past decade. As mentioned, distance learning can provide individuals in all settings with academic credentials and vocational and professional skills that can greatly enhance their career prospects. E-commerce opportunities abound; young people who pursue this option may have commercial dealings with individuals or companies all over the world but will often be able to receive professional training and conduct their business without having to relocate away from their families and support networks. At the grass-roots level, there is a growing number of ICT-related entrepreneurial opportunities for lower-income youth. One increasingly popular option for a young entrepreneur is to purchase a mobile phone through a microcredit programme and earn an income by providing low-cost phone services to others. ICT literacy, skills and accessibility are essential if young people are to use new technologies to take advantage of employment and entrepreneurial opportunities.

Large numbers of young people remain excluded from the information revolution; others are adversely affected by the ways in which the ICT revolution has challenged traditional forms of socialization. Many struggle to balance family and community influences with the global and cross-cultural influences of ICT. The increased use of mobile phones and the Internet has affected the daily interactions of youth almost everywhere. ICT can be a force for independence in the lives of young people, influencing behavioural and value patterns that differ from those of older generations. In this sense, ICT creates a new socialization landscape that in many ways challenges or erodes the traditional socialization process involving the transmission of long-established beliefs and practices through successive generations. The direction of socialization can even be reversed as the younger generation teaches the older generation about the uses and applications of emerging technologies. It is important to recognize, however, that ICT and the media do not preclude the continuing influence of such traditional actors as parents and schools in the socialization of children and youth. As further elaborated in the coming chapters, the emergence of a global media-driven youth culture propelled by ICT creates conditions for bidirectional socialization between generations. This challenges the common assumption that young people are not full members of society until they complete the process of socialization.

The next two chapters focus on various aspects of the emergence of a global media-driven youth culture. Chapter 5 begins with an introduction to youth cultures and examines the impact of new global media on the socialization of young people. It also explores the origins of new media, particularly as they tie in with young people's sociocultural status, and examines the need to provide young people with the tools they need to navigate their changing social environment. Chapter 6 focuses on how the new global media are affecting young people's roles in shaping their immediate societies. ●

Bibliography

British Broadcasting Corporation (no date). Commissioning (available from http://www.bbc.co.uk/commissioning/marketresearch/audiencegroup2.shtml).

Curtain, R. (2003). Promoting youth income generation opportunities through information and communication technologies (ICT): best practices in Asia and the Pacific; a 2003 update. Melbourne: Curtain Consulting.

European Commission (no date). Candidate countries Eurobarometer (available from http://europa.eu.int/comm/public_opinion/cceb_en.htm).

Mjaavatn, P.E. (1999). Modern lifestyle: a threat to young people's life. Tokyo: Child Research Net.

United Nations (2003a). *World Population Prospects: The 2002 Revision*; Highlights. ESA/P/WP.180.

_____ (2003b). *World Population Prospects: The 2002 Revision; Volume I*: Comprehensive Tables. Sales No. E.03.XIII.6.

_____ (2003c). *World Population Prospects: The 2002 Revision; Volume II: Sex and Age Distribution of the World Populations*. Sales No. E.03.XIII.7.

World Bank (2004). *World Development Indicators, 2004*. Washington, D.C.

World Health Organization (2004). *World Health Report, 2004: Changing History*. Geneva.

Chapter 5

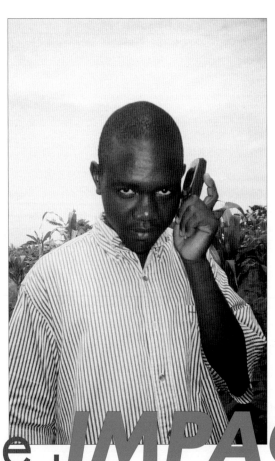

The **IMPACT** of global
media on youth culture

The increasingly widespread use of information and communication technology (ICT) must be viewed within the context of a much broader trend affecting the lives of young people today. The ongoing process of globalization is expanding the reach and influence of new technologies. It is becoming increasingly apparent that through modern-day media, ICT and global interconnectedness have combined very powerfully to influence the lives of young people, creating what is referred to here as a global media-driven youth culture.

WHAT IS YOUTH CULTURE?

Young people today are growing up in an increasingly commercialized, media-saturated world. In many ways, the concepts of "youth" as a distinct category and of a shared "youth culture" are relatively new, having emerged in the 1950s in the wake of the post-war expansion of consumerism in the Western world. Young people acquired greater spending power and were able to express their own wants and needs, and marketers increasingly began to target them with distinctive products such as youth-oriented music, fashion and media. Traditional youth cultures existed well before this time (Bennett, 2000); however, the modern media have reflected, and to some extent have produced, significant changes in both the socialization and sociocultural status of young people.

The concept of a "global youth culture" is not easy to define, as it reflects the implicit assumption that a majority of the world's young people share a common cultural framework. How can youth living under very different social conditions be incorporated into a unified cultural category? It is possible if the concept of youth culture is used to contextualize the lives of contemporary young people by acknowledging the combined or overlapping dimensions of personal and collective identity formation. In this sense, youth culture serves as a reference point for individuals developing their identity, very often while testing their ascribed roles at home, school and work. It is an unregulated area between the control and authority of the adult world and the freedom experienced among one's peers (Brake, 1980). In essence, youth culture can be interpreted as young people's own free space, which offers an alternative to the adult world as one develops, questions, and assumes roles in one's society.

In the late 1970s, researchers began examining youth in working-class subcultures and middle-class countercultures, both of which are cultures of consumption. There are also differentiated youth cultures with conscious group identities, connected with civic organizations or other articulated fields of operation such as non-governmental organizations (NGOs). Anti-consumerism movements represent a type of global youth culture in which the links between participants are based not on the consumption of particular products but on shared values and objectives such as promoting global democracy. By the late 1990s, it became natural for shared-value cultures to extend beyond national borders.

The various alternatives notwithstanding, youth cultures today tend to be strongly associated with commercialism—increasingly so as young people become more widely acknowledged as autonomous consumers and targeted by marketing campaigns. Superficial or not, a central feature of the global youth culture is that young people around the world are connected by their consumption of certain commercial products. Consequently, it is impossible to undertake an effective examination of youth cultures without exploring young people's relationship with the media. Global youth culture is created, adapted, accessed and disseminated largely through worldwide telecommunications networks that are rapidly expanding to reach many different parts of the world. The Internet, local and satellite television and radio, and other popular media are the channels through which youth-oriented cultural influences are transferred using music, direct advertising, websites and other means. Defined within this context, the current youth culture is clearly international in nature, as the consumption habits associated with it are to be found wherever young people have purchasing power.

Media and communication channels are being used to generate and strengthen new youth cultures centred around music, movie and sports stars, and around particular consumer goods and lifestyles; these cultural products have, in their own complex way, linked young people from all different countries and cultures and have produced a shared consciousness, leading to entirely new patterns and forms of socialization.

THE OLD AND NEW LANDSCAPE OF SOCIALIZATION

For young people, the traditional process of socialization involves gradually taking on the adult roles and responsibilities assigned to them by society. Developmental psychologists speak of certain developmental tasks with cognitive, affective and sexual dimensions that contribute to the formation of one's social, cultural and individual identity. Socialization entails becoming a more active, productive member of society, assuming the obligations of adulthood, becoming independent, and possibly leaving one's family home. In societies offering a formal education, this transition also involves achieving a relatively stable position in the education, housing, and labour markets. The more complex a society is, the more gradual, unclear and difficult this process becomes. The young people of today face many challenges in cobbling together a workable identity, a process many scholars refer to as "identity work" (Ziehe and Stubenrauch, 1982; Ziehe, 1992).

From a sociological perspective, socialization generally represents a process in which a younger member of a society or community adopts the values, norms and moral order of his or her group. In anthropology, this is often referred to as enculturation, or the process through which the cultural heritage of a society or community is passed on to its children and young people. Within these contexts, an individual is considered an adult when he or she has thoroughly internalized the prevailing values, or in other words, has been completely socialized.

In general terms, cultures may be classified as postfigurative, cofigurative or prefigurative (Mead, 1970). In a postfigurative culture socialization is straightforward and unidirectional, involving the transfer of basic values from the older to the younger generation. Such societies are often strict and authoritarian.

In a cofigurative culture, both children and adults also learn from their peers, though the direction of socialization is still from the older to the younger generation, configured so that the relationship between parents and children and between teachers and students is hierarchical. Various agents, including parents, extended family networks,

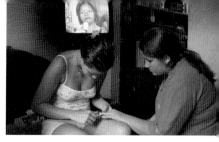

schools and other institutions, deliver a values package for children and young people to adopt. The succession of generations is seen as natural in the traditional model of socialization (Giddens, 1994). An important aspect of this relationship, as implied above, is the fact that the transfer of traditional symbols and practices from adults to children requires hierarchy. In such a setting, adults are capable of compelling children to conform to social and cultural demands and expectations. These circumstances are believed to be more typical of oral cultures, which anthropologists usually consider very traditional. In literate cultures, traditions tend to become thinner and weaken,[1] the succession of generations fractures, socialization becomes more complicated, and customary authority figures lose their hold on society's younger members.

In the traditional model of socialization, children and young people are regarded as subordinate to adults. In the contemporary interpretation, children and young people still learn important values from their elders and strengthen their socialization experience through peer interaction,[2] but they are also engaged in the transfer of knowledge to the older generation, as they have new skills and perspectives to share in evolving cultures. This prefigurative cultural framework features a two-directional process of socialization that often occurs when societies are changing rapidly and intergenerational roles and relationships are not as clearly defined. Arguably, these circumstances characterize many of today's societies, in which children and young people effectively grow up with new operational structures and measures of competence, often learned through the process of education and play. In some areas, the knowledge and skills of society's older members have become obsolete, and there are fields to which the younger members of a culture are almost by nature more receptive than their elders.

In many ways, the characteristics of a prefigurative culture are exemplified by the relationship between young people and the Internet, which (along with television) has played a major role in creating and perpetuating a global media culture. Young people are adept at both using the Internet and contributing to its content, which means that they are able to exercise some control over the very processes that are influencing their socialization.

There are a number of popular misconceptions surrounding young people's use of the Internet. Several theories suggest that children of the "information age" are micro-monsters and web sharks whose cognitive processes, hand-eye coordination and functional observation speed are such that their levels of ability and skill far surpass those of their parents and teachers (Tapscott, 1997). Furthermore, terms such as Generation@ or Net-Kids imply that virtually all young people are engaged in a broad range of ICT activities and that any disparity in the use of new technologies is above all a generational problem. However, the results of most empirical studies indicate that claims of a generational divide are exaggerated (Welling, 2003). Inequalities in ICT use appear to be more closely associated with income and educational factors; statistical evidence shows that young people who have little formal education and/or come from low-income households are less likely than their higher-income and more highly educated peers to be regular users of computers and the Internet (Welling, 2003).

Massive amounts of technology literature relating to online socialization and similar themes have been churned out.[3] However, the issues are almost always addressed from a theoretical perspective; consideration of what the Internet might represent in societal, social and cultural terms is lacking. Furthermore, the research field is characterized by fragmentation, small sample groups, non-comparability, and a Western cultural focus. Research has been conducted that extends beyond simple case studies, with qualitative and quantitative methods employed and both online and offline materials utilized; however, such research has not yet reached the level of cultural comparison. There is little empirical data indicating how young people really use the Internet and other forms of ICT in everyday life (Holloway and Valentine, 2003).

According to Paul Hodkinson (2003), who has researched the Internet forums of one youth subculture, net forums tend to strengthen existing strands of identity and pre-existing style-based subcultures. Young people who have access to the Internet seem to use it as part of their local socialization. They participate less often in so-called virtual communities, tending to do so only when they are driven by special interest in a site's programme (Hodkinson, 2003; Holloway and Valentine, 2003; Media Awareness Network, 2004).

In some contexts, the Internet may signify a dimension of identity and group belonging beyond one's immediate social environment; for young people in sparsely settled areas the Internet has global symbolic value (Laegran, 2002; 2003a; 2003b; Sharkey, 2002), and for young immigrants it may be a cross-border bridge-building place to maintain contact with their native cultures (Kinnunen, 2003). Research and theories concerning young people's relationship with the Internet have been criticized for making those who use it extensively sound like strange, perhaps exotic and weird creatures, somehow detached, floating through empty space in everyday social situations. The criticism relates to contextualization and demarcation; research tends to be focused on the way young people in such studies seem to be totally and excessively immersed either in virtual life on the Internet or in offline culture, with little effort made to analyse the interactions between these worlds (Hodkinson, 2003; Holloway and Valentine, 2003). The critique also concerns the scant attention generally paid in such research to the ways in which young people build their Internet-centred interactive culture in existing institutions such as the school and the family (Holloway and Valentine, 2003).

Identifying an aspect of the global media culture such as Internet use as part of a prefigurative, two-directional socialization process raises a series of questions: Into what are children and young people being socialized? What are the values, norms and moral structures of the global media culture into which they are being initiated? How does this socialization take place under conditions of rapid social change? The media culture context also raises an important question with regard to the direction and agents of socialization: If the global youth media culture is best defined as prefigurative (two-directional), what does this mean for tradition?

YOUTH CULTURES, PEER GROUPS AND SOCIALIZATION

The birth of youth cultures has been tied to the development of teen marketing (Brake, 1980). In today's world, peer groups and the products of the culture industry are contributing greatly to the evolution of youth culture; peer groups are becoming ever-stronger agents of socialization, and at times this creates conflict within the socialization process, as the role of parents and family has weakened in many contexts. The traditional roles and assumptions associated with the succession of generations and their inherent hierarchies have started to crumble. Socialization is no longer an automatic process in which adults simply transfer prevailing values to young people for their own use, as is the case with so-called direct socialization. In some settings, formal institutions have become more necessary; public, civic[4] and other organizations specializing in youth development have taken over some aspects of the socialization process, as parents, extended family members and neighbours can no longer manage on their own. For many, youth has come to signify a period during which young people are exposed to a multitude of influences and adopt values only through experimentation, with social values modified to such an extent that the whole society changes. Peer interaction has a surreptitious impact on socialization as young people experiment, investigate and test the principles, rules, customs, and habits of adult cultures outside the realm of adult influence.

The shift from traditional and controlled processes of socialization to more contemporary, two-directional socialization on a global scale has brought about a massive increase in the number of hybrid youth cultures. As mentioned previously, this process challenges and breaks down traditions and weakens the succession of generations; presently, the impact of these changes is most apparent in developing countries, where traditional socialization has maintained a strong foothold. It is important to recognize, however, that there are wide variations within and between countries; how adult relations with children and young people take shape in different cultures is often determined at the level of each community and society.

The emergence of the global media-driven youth culture signifies the building of a new landscape of socialization. With the structures and traditional roles of families undergoing major changes, youth cultures and youth media have emerged as entirely new agents of socialization, giving rise to new forms of socialization. One of the earliest examples is the student and youth movements of the 1960s, which had a major impact on popular culture. In some societies, the activities of this era brought about cultural change, including a rearrangement of relations between different age groups and generations and the breakthrough of the "consumer culture" mentality (Martin, 1981). In using the example of the student movements of the 1960s and the expressive revolution of the time, it is not implied that a global media-driven youth culture would give rise to the same sort of youth revolts in different countries. The point being made is that fundamental changes are taking place in the relationship between generations that have altered authority structures and the conditions of socialization in many societies.

THE INTERPLAY OF GLOBAL AND
LOCAL CULTURES AND SOCIALIZATION

One traditional feature of peer groups and youth cultures is that they are local by nature, which derives from the conventional assumption that interaction typically occurs face-to-face.[5] When this apparent axiom is considered within the modern context, it might be said that young users of media products have mediated relations within the global culture but that their peer groups are still local by nature. Local and global influences are not mutually exclusive; rather, the former may be understood as an aspect of the latter.

The previous section reviewed the changes in the conditions for socialization in many societies following the Second World War, indicating how young people's new relative autonomy in the use of their leisure time and the emergence of youth-focused marketing formed a free space and optimal conditions for the development of a youth culture. From the beginning, the youth movement and youth culture were perceived as subversive, as they challenged the system of education and other institutions symbolizing or promoting adulthood through their own (often ambivalent and politically unarticulated) forms of rebellion. Films, pop music and youth fashion have further defined this culture as distinct from the more general or traditional culture.

Media messages are not transmitted or received in a vacuum; people are surrounded by resources for specialized interpretation and operate within their own interpretive communities. Most people process information based on values, perspectives, opinions and modes of understanding acquired through early socialization, membership in social networks and personal experience, and this shapes their responses to media content. Even when people are exposed to subjects they know nothing about, their core beliefs and general orientations—or interpretive schema—will determine how they selectively assimilate and interpret the information (Curran, 2002). Global media have accelerated this assimilation process, but it is not new; historically, there have been some surprising and often complex reciprocities and interactions between countries around the world, the result of which has been the hybridization of both Western and non-Western cultures (Sreberny-Mohammadi, 1996). Cultural currents tend to be defined by certain features or qualities depending on the cultural landscape; global cultural currents tend to be multidirectional and highly variable and adaptive.

Successful global media marketers are able to distinguish and cater to the unique needs of various target audiences; they understand that they must adapt their products and services to local cultures in order to gain a foothold in local markets. Local and regional media markets are growing in Brazil, Egypt, India and Mexico, for example, with specialized content presented in different languages (Sinclair, Jacka and Cunningham, 1996). Whether or not media messages are adapted to suit particular audiences or presented in their original form, responses can vary widely. Local conditions and traditions always imprint incoming information, so messages may be met with a positive reaction, ambivalence, or even opposition and criticism. Soap operas, for example, can be interpreted differently by viewers from diverse national or ethnic backgrounds because they draw upon different belief systems and cultural references to make sense of media content (Curran, 2002). Much of what appears in the global media originates in the West, and

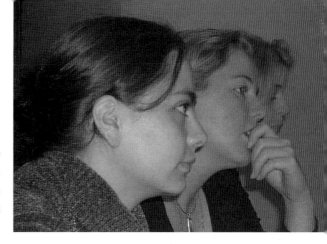

non-Western cultures have become actively selective and adaptive in their consumption, whether it is a question of television programmes, consumer goods, or thoughts and ideas. This type of two-directional interplay between local and global influences is reflected in the concept of "glocalization" (Robertson, 1994).

To sum up some of the major points made thus far, the emergence of a global media culture represents an extension of developments that have occurred over the past half-century—namely, the emergence of distinct youth cultures in the urbanized and industrialized areas of the world following the Second World War, the rising influence of peer groups and formal educational institutions, and the diminishing role of parents and community elders. Global media have come to constitute an independent and powerful agent of socialization for young people, and tensions have arisen as it has effectively challenged the more traditional agents of socialization.

In a contemporary interpretation of socialization, children and young people are seen as participants in the formation and maintenance of peer groups, and their interaction with one another produces a socializing effect. Through their membership in peer groups and shared youth cultures, young people have thus been able to contribute to their own socialization, and tools such as the Internet and other elements of the global media culture have reinforced this trend. These developments require serious, in-depth research before any pronouncements are made about whether they are positively or negatively affecting the lives of young people.

GLOBAL MEDIA AND THE SOCIOCULTURAL STATUS OF YOUNG PEOPLE

Within the ever-evolving global media context, the category of "youth" must be continuously reexamined. As the significance of age differences within the marketplace has increased, so have the designations applied to them. Marketers now use newly invented terms such as "tweenagers", "middle youth", "kidults" and "adultescents"—categories that intentionally blur the differences between children, youth and adults. The emergence of labels such as "Generation X" (and its subsequent mutations) reflects both the importance and the complexity of age-based distinctions in the contemporary media landscape (Ulrich and Harris, 2003).

"Youth" has become a symbolic value that can be marketed to a wide range of audiences; examples include the marketing of fashion products and make-up to young girls aspiring to escape the constraints of childhood, and the marketing of much contemporary rock music to adults aspiring to recover "lost" values of youthful energy and rebellion. In the increasingly competitive environment of contemporary media, such distinctions have a growing commercial significance. How old you are—or how old you imagine yourself to be—is increasingly defined by what you consume. Youth culture, it would seem, is no longer just for young people.

Global media products and globally recognized brands are a crucial dimension of young people's identity formation worldwide; however, as mentioned, they are not consumed in a vacuum. A common presumption is that the pressures of global marketing are leading to a kind of homogenization, in which cultural specificities are all but effaced. This fails to take into account that youth culture is a local as well as a global phenomenon (Nayak, 2003). Young people use, adapt and interpret global products in unique ways based on their own local cultures and experiences; in the process, they create "hybrid" cultural forms whose meanings vary according to local and national circumstances. For example, hip-hop music may have originated in the United States, but it has come to mean something different as it has been appropriated and (increasingly) produced in France, Germany and South Africa (Bennett, 2000).

Because global media developments tend to have such a powerful impact on young people, it is worth taking a closer look at the changing nature of contemporary media and to consider the implications of its new forms.

THE CHANGING NATURE OF CONTEMPORARY MEDIA

Much of the discourse on young people and the media is polarized. On the one hand, there is the idea that childhood, as traditionally defined, is dying or disappearing, and that the media are primarily to blame. It has been observed that it was the printing press that effectively created the concept of childhood, and television has destroyed it (Postman, 1983). Some scholars point to the demise of children's traditional games and distinctive styles of dress; the increasing homogenization of young people's and adults' leisure pursuits, language, eating habits and tastes in entertainment; and the increase in youth crime, drug-taking, sexual activity and teenage pregnancy—all of which, it is argued, can be traced to the influence of the media. Further reference is made to the erotic use of children in commercials and movies, the prevalence of "adult" themes in young people's books, and what is seen as the misguided emphasis on children's rights (Postman, 1983).

On the other hand, media are also seen as a liberating force for young people, creating a new "electronic generation" that is more open, democratic, and socially aware than previous generations. In this context, the Internet is seen as having given young people "powerful new tools for enquiry, analysis, self-expression, influence and play"; as a result, members of the "net generation" are "hungry for expression, discovery and their own self-development" (Tapscott, 1997, p. 5). Rap music, talk shows and cable television, along with the Internet, are seen as examples of the "great creative explosions of modern culture", and it is argued that they represent a growing, and welcome, challenge to centralized adult control (Katz, 1997).

There may be some truth in each of these perspectives, but it may also be argued that both overestimate the power of the media and underestimate the ambivalent and contradictory nature of contemporary social change. To regard young people as *either* passive victims of, *or* somehow liberated by, the media is to grossly oversimplify the process. It is possible to gain a better understanding of the changing nature of the modern media and its relevance to youth by exploring several different aspects of the issue using a more multifaceted approach. In the subsections below, technologies, economics, texts and audiences are given separate consideration; in each of these areas, young people have been among the avant-garde in many contemporary developments.

Changing technologies

In many countries in both the developed and developing world, the most critical aspect of the recent changes in media technologies is their proliferation.[6] The household television screen has become the delivery point for a growing range of media and means of distribution. The number of channels has grown, both on terrestrial television and (more spectacularly) with the advent of cable, satellite and digital technologies; the screen is also being used for video in various forms, as well as for an ever-broadening range of digital media and products including computer games, CD-ROMs and the Internet.

There has been a convergence between information, communication, and media technologies, made possible by digitization; like the other developments identified here, this process has been commercially driven. Digital television, Internet set-top boxes, online shopping, video-on-demand and other developments are increasingly blurring the distinctions between linear broadcast or "narrowcast" media such as television and interactive media such as the Internet.

These and other developments have made media technologies more accessible. Media products that were once prohibitively expensive, as well as a wide range of new media forms and options, have been brought within the reach of the domestic consumer. The retail price of video camcorders, digital cameras and multimedia personal computers (PCs) has steadily fallen as their capabilities have increased. In principle, at least, the Internet represents a means of communication and distribution that—unlike many earlier media forms—is not exclusively controlled by a small elite. With the exponential increase in users and applications, it is argued, the boundaries between production and consumption, and between mass communication and interpersonal communication, are beginning to break down.

These changes have several implications for young people. Families with children constitute a very receptive, and therefore important, market for new media technologies. Cable and satellite television programming has been strongly targeted towards younger audiences, and much of the advertising and promotion for home computers trades on the popular mystique surrounding young people's natural affinity for technology (Nixon, 1998). The take-up of satellite and cable television, video, camcorders and home computers is often proportionally much higher in households with children than in those without. Greater access to an ever-widening range of media technology options has been accompanied by increased individualization and personalization in their application. Young people, particularly in rich developed countries, are now likely to live in households with two or more television sets; in the United Kingdom, three quarters of teenagers now have televisions in their bedrooms, and almost half have video cassette recorders.

While collective uses of the media, particularly "family viewing", have far from disappeared, there has been a marked trend towards more independent usage, encouraged by the general democratization of relationships within the family and the relaxation of parental authority (Livingstone and Bovill, 1999). Young people's increased access to various media has generated growing concern about their exposure to violence, pornography, and other material hitherto largely confined to the domain of adults. In many instances, this has led to calls for stricter regulation and censorship; the creation of the V-chip and content-blocking software reflects the search for a "technological fix".[7]

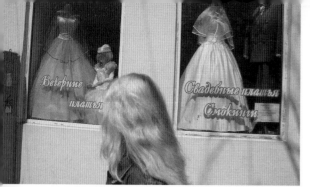

While new media technologies and their use have been characterized by explosive growth, the scale of these developments should not be exaggerated. Levels of access will certainly increase significantly in the coming years as prices continue to fall, yet there is also a growing polarization between the "technology rich" and the "technology poor". In most countries, Internet users tend to have relatively high levels of education and income. In Bulgaria, the poorest 65 per cent of the population account for only 29 per cent of Internet users. In Chile, 89 per cent of Internet users have a tertiary education; the corresponding figures are 65 per cent for Sri Lanka and 70 per cent for China (United Nations Development Programme, 2001). In the United Kingdom, fewer than half as many working-class children as middle-class children have access to a PC at home, and only one tenth as many are linked to the Internet (Livingstone and Bovill, 1999). As true today as it was in the 1950s with the advent of television, those with more disposable income are almost always the early adopters of new technologies; they have newer and more powerful equipment, and more opportunities to develop the skills and competencies needed to use it. Economic considerations are particularly important in developing countries, where a large majority of young people do not have computers or Internet access, mainly for financial reasons; buying a computer and getting "wired to the Web" are still big investments in many countries. Poor infrastructure puts young people in smaller towns and villages at a further disadvantage. Technical problems can discourage widespread Internet use in some countries and can prevent young people from fully appreciating or taking advantage of all the possibilities the Web offers. Apart from these considerations, there are also young people who shy away from the Internet because of the prevalence of English-language content, or more to the point, the absence of content in their own language (Gigli, 2004).

The various limitations notwithstanding, new technologies and many of the cultural forms made possible by them are typically identified with the young. Computer games are predominantly aimed at the youth market, and popular music (particularly dance music) is increasingly being generated by digital technology using sampling, editing and other software. In Australia, young people between the ages of 18 and 24 are five times more likely to be Internet users than are those over the age of 55. In Chile, 74 per cent of users are under 35 years old, and in China the corresponding share is 84 per cent; other countries follow the same pattern (Gigli, 2004). The growing accessibility of ICT (especially new media technologies) is enabling some young people to play a more active role as cultural producers. In the wealthier population sectors, more and more teenagers have home computers in their bedrooms that can be used to create music, manipulate images and edit video to a relatively professional standard.

Changing economics

The technological developments reviewed thus far have both contributed to and been reinforced by fundamental economic changes in the media industries. These changes are part of a much larger trend towards the development of a global free market economy. Reforms such as economic liberalization and the privatization of State-owned enterprises are at the centre of this historic shift, particularly in developing countries. The telecommunications and broadcasting sectors have been among the early targets in the restructuring of public services and State industries in many countries (Petrazzini, 1995).

Recent developments such as these in both developed and developing countries point to the growing privatization of the media and the relative decline in public sector service provision in the relevant sectors. The large majority of media forms and outlets are commercially driven; even those that initially were not, such as the Internet, are increasingly subject to commercial imperatives, such as the need to carry advertising.Technological convergence has been mirrored by economic convergence, as large media conglomerates have flourished under the liberalization policies of many national Governments. Meanwhile, in settings in which the State remains involved in this realm of activity, public sector service provision has gradually been commercialized from within, and regulation concerning the social and cultural functions of the media is gradually being abandoned.

One inevitable consequence of media commercialization has been the integration of media industries. The media market is now dominated by a small number of transnational conglomerates; for nationally based companies, success in the international market has become a necessity for survival. Many of today's largest cable and satellite companies have a stake in a number of sizeable world markets, including Europe and the United States. Significantly, most of these corporations are cross-media conglomerates; they integrate broadcasting, publishing, digital technology, and other aspects of media-focused ICT, and in many cases are involved in both hardware and software industries. Vertical integration has thus been achieved through a form of horizontal integration. However, integration does not necessarily mean homogenization; growing competition has led to the fragmentation of audiences and the rise of niche marketing. Media and media products are increasingly being targeted towards specialized segments of the mass audience, albeit on a global scale.

These developments are affecting young people in a number of different ways, some of them ambiguous. In the contemporary era of niche marketing, young people have become an increasingly valuable market, not only because they have their own disposable income, but also because of their ability to set trends and influence other consumers. For example, cable television offers a plethora of specialized channels competing to attract youth audiences, and on both terrestrial and non-terrestrial channels there has been a significant increase in the amount (though not necessarily in the quality or diversity) of material and airtime targeted at young people.

Integrated marketing has become an almost indispensable aspect of media directed at young people. Television programmes are tied in with films, CDs, comics and computer games — not to mention T-shirts, posters, food and drink, and a multitude of other products. One of the most successful schemes to emerge in this context is the cross-media franchise, in which the identity of the "original" text is far from clear; media commodities are packaged and marketed as integrated phenomena, rather than the text coming first and the merchandising following later. These developments are particularly apparent in mainstream popular music.

Despite such efforts, a significant proportion of commercial products aimed at young people fail to generate a profit; the market is more competitive and therefore more uncertain. Within such a milieu, there is some justification in producers' recurrent claim that young people are a volatile, complex market that cannot easily be defined or controlled.

Changing texts

The developments described here are perhaps most obviously manifested in the changing characteristics of media texts. Here, too, there has been a significant degree of convergence, both between texts themselves and between media. The distinctions between video products, computer games, movies, television shows, advertisements and print texts have become increasingly irrelevant, and more and more media texts are spin-offs of or tie-ins with other texts or commodities. While this may be most evident in developed countries, such convergence is spreading to other parts of the world through global marketing campaigns and the advancement and diversification of satellite technology (Volkmer, no date).

Intertextuality has become a dominant characteristic of contemporary media. Many of the texts that are perceived as distinctively postmodern are highly allusive, self-referential and ironic. They self-consciously draw upon other texts in the form of pastiche, homage or parody; they juxtapose incongruous elements from different historical periods, genres or cultural contexts; and they play with established conventions of form and representation. In the process, they implicitly address their readers or viewers as knowing, "media literate" consumers.

Many of these new media forms are characterized by interactivity. Some of the more enthusiastic advocates of interactive multimedia see them as a means of liberation from the constraints of more traditional linear media such as film and television; hypertext, CD-ROMs and computer games are seen to blur or even eliminate the distinction between "reader" and "writer". In recent years, interactivity appears to have become an increasingly important characteristic even of the mainstream media, as clearly demonstrated by the success of so-called reality television.

Many of these developments are dictated primarily by economic considerations. Pastiche and parody often serve as little more than window dressing for media that are in all other respects highly conventional. It could even be argued that irony has become just another marketing device, enabling media corporations to secure additional profit by recycling existing properties. Likewise, intertextuality can be seen as a consequence of increasing commodification and the need to exploit successes across a wider range of media on a shorter time scale. Further, despite the potential for interactivity, there is an undeniable gap between rhetoric and reality in a great deal of commercial software; many so-called interactive texts are far from interactive, offering a fixed and highly circumscribed repertoire of possibilities.

Many of the features and characteristics described above apply particularly to media texts that are aimed at, or are most popular with, young people. Many of the most innovative new cultural forms have initially been targeted at this audience, reaching the adult market somewhat later. There is clear evidence of the trends described here in, for example, the ironic, self-conscious intertextuality of contemporary comics; the use of sampling in rap and dance music; the allusive, montage-based style of music videos; the convergence of music, visual arts and electronic media in club culture; and the genuinely interactive and highly complex nature of some computer games. It is important to note, however, that for all the inflated rhetoric surrounding "cyberculture", there have been some highly innovative uses of the Internet among a small minority of young people that genuinely do point to its emergence as a distinctive cultural form.

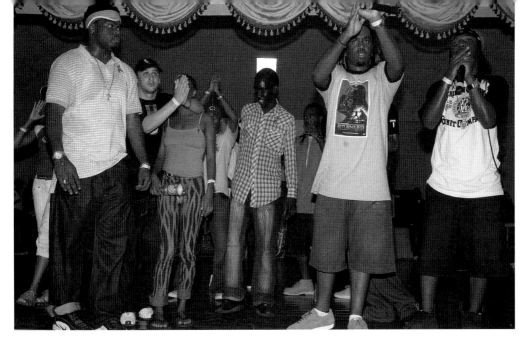

Finally, mention must be made of important changes at the level of content; it is developments in this area that often cause the most alarm among adult critics. In many countries, children's television has undergone a steady transformation over the past 20 years and now incorporates topics that would once have been considered taboo, such as sex, drugs and family breakdown. Likewise, magazines and books aimed at the early-teenage market have attracted widespread criticism for their frank and explicit treatment of such issues (Rosen, 1997). There is also, increasingly, a degree of subversiveness and cynicism apparent in mainstream popular culture, as evidenced by the content of various youth-oriented cartoons that have been launched in recent years.[8] Such cartoons are permeated with references to other texts and genres, sometimes in the form of direct quotations or "sampling". They raid existing cultural resources, borrowing from both the high culture and the popular culture of the past and present in a fragmentary and often apparently parodic manner. Comparing current animation series with those of 30 years ago, one is struck not only by the much faster pace of the former, but also by their irony and intertextuality, and by the complex interplay between reality and fantasy; these factors are characteristic of postmodern texts (Wells, 2002). Their ability to disturb more conservative adult commentators appears to derive, at least in part, from the fact that they contain "adult" content in a genre that is traditionally associated with children.

Changing audiences

The new media environment presupposes quite different kinds of competence and knowledge — and might be seen to encourage very different forms of "activity" — among audiences. Contemporary media are increasingly addressing young people as highly "media literate" consumers. Whether they actually are more media literate, and what this term actually means, are issues that require careful consideration.

Although it is frequently claimed that ICT/media-related developments are creating a wider range of choices for consumers, this assertion is only partly true. The proliferation of television channels has led to a significant increase in the quantity of programming available, even taking into account that much of it is repeated. On one level, these developments clearly do empower audiences to schedule their own viewing, at least within the range of material available; however, they also raise some awkward questions about how viewers locate and select what they want to watch. Once again, there is the issue of the skills and competencies young people require to effectively navigate and evaluate the increased content being made available.

The dramatic increase in options appears to be contributing to the fragmentation of audiences, as media are increasingly targeted at, and their products marketed to, specialized groups of consumers. The increasingly affordable access to enormous numbers of television channels through cable, satellite and other service providers may bring about a decline in general audience broadcasting (and the "common culture" that makes it possible) in favour of "narrowcasting". The Internet is perhaps the best and most promising medium for those with specialized or minority interests.

One factor to consider in relation to these issues is, again, interactivity. Leaving aside the question of whether surfing the Internet actually is more "active" than surfing television channels or browsing through a magazine, there are some important questions about whether audiences actually want greater activity. The Internet may allow users much greater control over the selection of content and the pace at which it is perused; however, it also permits much more detailed surveillance of consumer behaviour. It is now very easy to track users' movements within and between particular websites and thereby build up consumer profiles that can subsequently become the basis for targeted electronic advertising.

While the eventual outcomes of these developments are difficult to predict, it is clear that young people in all parts of the world are regarded by many in the media industries as being at the forefront of change, largely owing to the natural evolution of young people's place in modern society, but also, perhaps, as a consequence of having been placed in such a position by the operations of the market. Young people are encouraged to be "early adopters" and may perhaps serve as an indication of what is likely to occur within the general population. In several respects, young people's uses of media do seem to be characterized by increasing choice, interactivity and diversity-even if these opportunities are not equally available to all.

The consequences and implications of these changes have been interpreted in sharply contrasting ways. In the English-speaking world, at least, sensational stories about the harm allegedly inflicted on young people by the media are increasingly dominating the headlines. The furor surrounding the influence of video games following the massacre at Columbine High School[9] is only one recent example of the recurrent moral panics that have come to characterize public debate. Various segments of the media routinely and uncritically recycle examples of astonishingly weak research purporting to show, for example, that large numbers of children are busily swapping computer-generated pornography on the playground, or that young people are being encouraged to commit car thefts as a result of their exposure to video games. The view of the media as an essentially corrupting influence has a very long history (Barker and Petley, 2001).

While the public debate has increasingly centred around shielding young people from harm, reflecting a kind of moral protectionism, the discourses that circulate within the media industries seem to be moving in an entirely different direction. In the latter context, young people are no longer seen as innocent and vulnerable to influence, but are increasingly regarded as sophisticated, demanding, media-wise consumers. Attempts to protect young people and to educate them through media such as television have increasingly been condemned as paternalistic and patronizing. Adults, it is argued, have been talking down to them for far too long. There are those who contend that in this new market-led environment, young people are at last being empowered to make their own decisions about what they will experience and learn about, without the controlling hand of adults who profess to know what is good for them. These discursive changes clearly reflect broader changes in the status of young people as a distinct social group. However, there is often a fundamental blurring or confusion between the notion of young people as potential or actual citizens and the notion of young people as consumers.

BLURRING BOUNDARIES AND THE AMBIGUITIES SURROUNDING YOUTH

Broadly speaking, it is possible to discern two sets of forces at play in the developments that have been described. One is that the boundaries between young people and adults appear to be blurring. To a much greater extent than traditional broadcast television, the newer media such as video, the Internet, and cable and satellite technologies allow young people access to material previously restricted to adults (Postman, 1983). Youth are increasingly addressed as autonomous consumers who are encouraged to make their own decisions about what they will buy, watch and read. Via the Internet, they can communicate much more easily with each other and with adults, without even having to identify themselves as young people. Even in the material produced explicitly for them, there are manifestations of aspects of the world that were previously considered unsuitable for them to see or to know about.

As noted previously, "youth" has become an extremely elastic category that seems to be extending ever further upward (Frith, 1993). In their shared enthusiasm for certain kinds of music, sportswear or video games, for example, 10-year olds and 40-year olds may be seen as members of a "youth" market that is quite self-consciously distinct from the "family" market. In this environment, "youth" has come to be perceived as a lifestyle choice that is defined by its relationship to specific brands and commodities and that is also available to those who fall well outside its biological limits (which are fluid in any case). For the producers and distributors of media products such as youth television and popular music, "youth" possesses a symbolic significance that may be linked as much to fantasy identities as to material possibilities—a phenomenon that serves to widen the audience and thus enhance its market value.

While some boundaries are becoming blurred, others are becoming more strongly defined. With young people's increased access to media technology, they no longer have to watch or read what their parents choose. As the youth niche market grows in importance, young people are increasingly able to confine themselves to media that are produced specifically for them. The new, postmodern cultural forms that characterize contemporary youth culture are in many respects highly exclusive of adults; they require particular cultural competencies and a prior knowledge of specific media texts (or in other words, a form of media literacy) only available to the young. While youth around the world are increasingly sharing a global media culture with one another, they appear to be sharing less and less with their own parents.

The ambiguity characterizing these developments reflects broader ambiguities in the social status of young people. They are becoming empowered both as citizens and as consumers, yet their own expressions of their needs are largely confined to the services or products adults can provide. In debates about the changing nature of schooling, leisure provision or the media, their voices are still rarely heard. Meanwhile, young people's leisure activities are steadily becoming more privatized and commercialized. More of their time is spent in unsupervised activity of some kind, and the cultural goods and services they consume increasingly have to be paid for in hard cash. One inevitable consequence of this is a rise in inequality between young people in both the social and media contexts. The polarization between rich and poor is positively reinforced by the commercialization of the media and the decline in public sector provision. Young people living in disadvantaged economic circumstances simply have less access to media goods and services; they live not only in different social worlds, but in different media worlds as well. One scholar has noted that "if globalization is a process of accelerated flow of media content, to most African cultures and children, it is also a process of accelerated exclusion".[10]

Overall, however, it may be concluded that many opportunities for creative development and expression and for social integration and democratization have evolved out of the advances made in this field; particularly important is the potential they offer for young people to become media producers in their own right. New technologies bring hitherto inaccessible means of cultural expression and communication within the reach of young people and enable them to disseminate their views and perspectives much more widely. Far from contributing to social polarization, the media can be a means of enabling young people to communicate across their differences. However, these developments will not take place automatically, or simply because the appropriate equipment is available. As a few selected case studies show, concerted and creative interventions will be needed at the level of social and cultural policy if young people's rights and capabilities as producers and consumers of electronic media are to be more fully realized.

MEDIA PROVISION: MUSIC VIDEO, NEWS AND ONLINE CULTURE

Media provision through music video

Music video, which is often hailed as an essentially youthful media form, can be seen as emblematic of several of the changes outlined in the first part of this chapter. Music video was among the first media genres to explore the potential of new technological developments such as digital editing and image manipulation. Economically, it typifies the global multimedia synergy that characterizes modern media industries. Textually, it is often seen to reflect a distinctively postmodern aesthetic characterized by allusion, pastiche and play. In addition, it has increasingly reflected the fragmentation of contemporary media audiences into specialized "taste communities".

Popular music never has been just about the music; today, it is part of a global commercial enterprise that integrates a wide range of media forms, including not only CDs and live events, but also radio, television, movies and magazines, as well as extensive secondary merchandising. In this context, every text effectively becomes a potential advertisement for other texts.

Music video emerged as an important marketing tool during the 1980s (*see box 5.1*), though the use of visual imagery in popular music originated much earlier, dating back at least to the visual jukeboxes of the 1940s (Shuker, 2001). There is also a tradition of

Box 5.1

THE MTV GENERATION

Music television entered a new era with the advent of the cable channel MTV in 1981. Owned by the media giant Viacom, based in the United States, MTV quickly became a leading force in the music industry.[a] During the 1990s, it began to export its programming globally via channels such as MTV Europe and MTV Asia, and while these channels observed set quotas for local performers, there was some resistance to the pan-continental approach. MTV Europe has since fragmented into a series of national channels that have local presenters and more targeted local programming, pointing to some of the potential limits to globalization, at least in the realm of music. In 2004, Viacom acquired a controlling interest in VIVA Media AG, its German equivalent, making Viacom the largest music television provider in the European heartland. In November of that year, MTV announced that it would begin broadcasting in Africa, which would allow it to reach the world's last major populated area not previously served by this network.

MTV has worked closely with major recording labels, not just selecting material to be aired but also influencing some of the content. Commercially, it has succeeded by targeting a valuable youth and young adult demographic that is more difficult for advertisers to reach through mainstream television. The network's early business model was premised on the fact that recording companies were paying for the programming (since the videos were effectively advertisements for their products).

The growth of MTV has not been without its problems. Competition from other music channels in the late 1980s compelled the network to retrench and diversify. Claiming that the music video format had grown stale, MTV began producing other types of programming, including "news", documentaries, animation, and dating game shows. With the emergence of more specialized music channels for the older, more mainstream market, MTV has also established subsidiary channels broadly covering dance, urban and alternative genres.

Initial academic responses to MTV celebrated its apparent blurring of the boundaries between image and reality, its reliance on intertextuality and pastiche, its disruption of conventional narrative norms, and its construction of a "decentred" or "fragmented" spectator.[b] Perhaps paradoxically, some of these observations coincided with those of more conservative critics, who saw MTV as the embodiment of an apolitical, amoral universe in which traditional humanist values and forms of rationality had effectively been abandoned.

More recent criticism reflects a significant tempering of these arguments.[c] A close look at today's music videos reveals that a large majority contain familiar settings, moods and themes, and fall within a limited range of predictable genres. Aside from performance-based pieces, most are concerned with conventional themes such as sexual relationships, growing up, fantasy and, to a limited extent, social issues. Furthermore, the apparent heterogeneity and incoherence of the imagery is often "anchored" or contained by the more conventional form of the music; the music makes sense of the images, pulling them back towards traditional forms of narrative or argument.

Nevertheless, it would be wrong to underestimate the potential for innovation and experimentation in music video, or its influence on a wide range of other media forms. To some degree, music video requires, and is possibly helping to cultivate, a new form of media literacy that poses new cognitive and emotional challenges. It presupposes the ability of consumers to process images and sounds at considerable speed, to tolerate ambiguity, and to interpret visual symbolism-which is qualitatively different from the media orientation of older generations.

[a] J. Banks, *Monopoly Television: MTV's Quest to Control the Music* (Boulder, Colorado: Westview Press, 1996).

[b] E.A. Kaplan, *Rocking Around the Clock: Music Television, Postmodernism, and Consumer Culture* (London: Methuen, 1987).

[c] A. Goodwin, *Dancing in the Distraction Factory: Music Television and Popular Culture* (London: Routledge, 1992).

movie musicals, dance movies and soundtracks, and many of the most successful contemporary films have music video spin-offs. Mainstream television has had a more ambiguous relationship with popular music. While the television industry has always been comfortable with family-friendly entertainment, it has often sought to tame or steer clear of the potentially "dangerous" aspects of popular music-such as implicit sexuality, rebellious-ness and violence-that are central to its appeal for youth audiences. Mainstream television has also found it difficult to cater to the more specialized and diverse tastes that have become increasingly important in popular music over the past two decades.

Music video provides a symptomatic indication of several broader tendencies within contemporary youth media. Its success clearly reflects the increasing importance of media, especially visual media, in youth culture. However, it also raises the question of who "owns" youth culture. To what extent is youth culture produced by young people themselves or merely produced for them by the multinational media industries? Large conglomerates have acted as gatekeepers, playing a powerful role in determining the kinds of music distributed, yet in an increasingly competitive environment their capacity to control the market is quite limited. Although music industry profits are substantial, a large majority of what is produced fails to generate sufficient revenues to cover costs. One of the key commodities in youth culture is authenticity, and much of the criticism of popular music among fans and commentators is directed against material seen to be too commercial or "fake". The music industry works hard to manage commercial risk, but the behaviour of consumers is far from predictable. In this area, as in other areas of youth culture, there is an ongoing struggle between the imperatives of capital and the needs and desires of audiences.

Media provision through news

Young people's interest in news media varies greatly around the world. In some countries, a substantial number of young people are attracted by the largely political fare of international public radio networks such as the British Broadcasting Corporation, Voice of America, Deutsche Welle, and Radio France Internationale. Survey findings indicate that in 2003, 16 per cent of young people between the ages of 15 and 19 listened to international radio in Albania; the corresponding proportions were 12 per cent in Bangladesh, 21 per cent in Nigeria, and 26 per cent in urban areas of Haiti (Gigli, 2004). In other countries, such as the United States, there has been a steep decline among youth in the readership of broadsheet newspapers and the viewership of flagship television news programmes, and the effects of these trends are compounded by what some critics see as the growing interest of young people in tabloid news, a genre frequently condemned for its preoccupation with sensationalism and its lack of serious political information (Times Mirror Center for the People and the Press, 1990). Similar trends have been noted in South Africa and the United Kingdom, where young people's interest in news media is minimal, particularly when it comes to media coverage of political affairs.[11]

While these findings may be seen as symptomatic of young people's broader cynicism about politics, they also highlight one of the largest problems with regard to media rights for youth, namely the lack of coverage of children and young people in the news. It has been noted that what little coverage there is of young people is very often characterized by sensationalism, highlighting child abuse, exploitation and violence, with scant

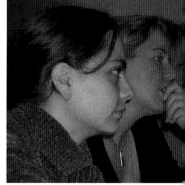

opportunity for young people to speak for themselves. Young people tend to feel excluded from or disserved by the media when they are portrayed simplistically as superficial, apathetic, poverty stricken, victimized or delinquent (Gigli, 2004).

Some critics suggest that young people are actively excluded from the domain of politics, and from the major public forums of political discourse, including the news media. They argue that mainstream news journalism has failed to keep pace with the changing cultural competencies of young people, that youth have a very different orientation towards information from that of older generations, and that they prefer the more informal and ironic style of digital media to the monotonously reassuring voice of conventional news journalism (Katz, 1993). From this perspective, it is the failure of the established news media to connect with the forms of everyday politics most important for this generation that accounts for the loss of younger audiences.

An analysis of news programmes produced specifically for young people in the United States and the United Kingdom revealed much about the critical responses of this group to television programming (Buckingham, 2000). The study examined two types of news programmes directed at youth. One type was very similar to the mainstream news in terms of style and presentation format but was aimed at making news accessible to a younger audience. This entailed some departures from the conventions of mainstream news, including adjustments in the balance between "foreground" and "background", the kind of language used, and the manner of presentation. To some extent this might be regarded as superficial window dressing, though some of the programmes also used young people as interviewers (albeit in a rather limited way) and included a viewers' access slot.

The programmes examined within this first category introduced some innovations but did not significantly challenge the status quo or what was seen to count as news. By contrast, the other types of programmes examined in the study departed more radically from the conventions of the genre. These were essentially news magazines and covered issues featured in the mainstream news and debated within the formal political domain. However, they offered a distinctly different conception of what might count as news and what form it might take. These programmes were characterized by a unique visual style and, at a more substantive level, reflected young people's own perspectives and concerns, not least because youth were recruited to write and present their own items.

The young people interviewed for the study preferred the more innovative and informal approach of the second type of programming. They found it important that these programmes did not talk down to their audiences. Young viewers also applauded the fact that the preferred programmes presented new information rather than just simplified versions of the mainstream news. There was considerable importance attached to graphics, camera work and editing, as well as to the focus on ordinary young people and attempts to present a young person's point of view (Buckingham, 2000).

Young people are very sensitive to age differences and are scathing in their criticism of programmes that appear to underestimate them. They also want programmes relevant to their everyday concerns, which are largely marginalized in the mainstream news. There is a real need for innovation if news is to reawaken the interest not only of younger audiences but of a large majority of other viewers as well. This is partly a

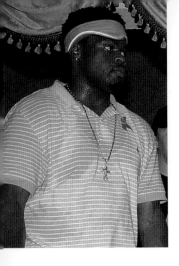

matter of developing new formal strategies, but it also requires a more fundamental rethinking of what is seen to count as news in the first place. The deferential stance that is invited and encouraged by mainstream news formats needs to be abandoned in favour of an approach that invites scepticism and active engagement. Much greater effort must be made not only to explain the causes and contexts of news events, but also to enable viewers to perceive the relevance of these events to their own everyday lives. News providers can no longer afford to confine their coverage to the words and actions of the powerful, or to the narrow and exclusive discourses that currently dominate the public sphere of social and political debate.

The avoidance of entertainment in favour of a narrow insistence on seriousness and formality in the dominant forms of news production systematically alienates younger audiences. Addressing this issue involves more than simply sugar-coating the pill, however. News providers could learn a great deal from the genres that are most successful in engaging younger audiences, perhaps taking some cues from MTV. Obviously, some of the more modern approaches can be a recipe for superficiality, but they can also offer news providers creative new ways to fulfil their mission to educate and inform-areas in which they have lost their edge, particularly among young people.

Media provision through online culture

The debate over the role of the Internet in young people's lives is often sharply polarized. Many regard this new medium primarily in terms of the potential risks. There is a high level of public anxiety about the accessibility of pornography on the Internet, and about the dangers of young people being seduced by online paedophiles or political extremists. There is also growing concern about the practice of online marketing to young people both through direct selling and through the gathering of market research data (Montgomery, 1997; Seiter, 2004). However, as mentioned in an earlier section within the context of two-directional socialization, the Internet can also be seen as a means of liberation and expression for young people. Chat groups, electronic mail and web pages represent avenues of autonomous creative expression and offer arenas in which, arguably, children and young people are no longer constrained by the limitations of their parents' cultures (Tapscott, 1997).

To what extent are such claims regarding the creativity and creative potential of online culture justified? As previously noted, much of the data presented here are fragmentary and anecdotal; leaving aside those using e-mail and instant messaging, the number of young people who could reasonably be regarded as active participants in online culture is relatively small. Much of the research in the field, including, for example, that on electronic fanzines (Leonard, 1998) or multi-user domains (Turkle, 1995), actually relates to young adults (those over the age of 18). Such research is almost bound to focus on unrepresentative cases; some of it appears unduly preoccupied with the more avant-garde manifestations of cyberculture. A crucial task for researchers at this stage is to consider how representative the early adopters might be, and to examine and analyse the more banal, everyday uses of these media.

Another important consideration is that researchers in this area are dealing with forms and aspects of the youth culture to which it is very difficult to gain access—and which, in many respects, seem almost deliberately designed to exclude them. Serious ethical dilemmas inevitably arise in this kind of research, particularly given the ease with which one can eavesdrop on apparently private communications, and these may be particularly acute in relation to young people.

Nevertheless, some researchers have provided illuminating case studies that are suggestive of some of the broader issues at stake. Home pages produced by young people on the World Wide Web, for example, have been interpreted in analyses as instances of "identity construction" analogous to the decoration of bedroom walls (Chandler and Roberts-Young, 1998). The home page is seen here as a hybrid form that combines aspects of public communication (such as broadcasting or publishing) and private communication (such as a personal diary or letter), and to some extent crosses the boundary between them. This hybridity is reflected particularly in the combination of written, verbal and visual forms of communication and expression that characterize these new media (Abbott, 1998). For some, the constant changes being made to the home pages of children and young people are symptomatic of a postmodern fluidity of identity; others have argued that the Internet is a place where young people feel they can be "truly themselves" (Tobin, 1998).

A related theme in this context is that of pedagogy. Some scholars argue that online communication produces "learning communities" that cross the boundaries of age and geography, and that are more democratic and collaborative than those of traditional educational institutions (Tobin, 1998). The relatively recent phenomenon of blogs (web logs) is seen to have particularly strong potential for promoting student-centred learning (Oravec, 2003) and providing opportunities for political activism among young people (Cushion, 2004; Kahn and Kellner, 2004). As in more general assertions about online communities, such arguments tend to neglect the occasionally undemocratic and exclusionary nature of some online communication. Nonetheless, the opportunities these media present for group interaction in comparison with equivalent older technologies such as the telephone are far superior.

The interactive and pedagogical aspects are particularly apparent in analyses of online fan cultures. Engaging in a unique form of "textual poaching" (Jenkins, 1992), fans of religious media texts explore and extend the pleasure they derive from them by reworking the texts through writing, song, artwork and other means (Flench, 1999). There is often an effort made to honour the original text by remaining as true to it as possible; for example, the fine details of the appearance or behaviour of a character may be replicated. In some cases, however, the original text is dramatically altered or adapted to reflect the particular interests of fans or fan groups. Fan sites and "web rings" often develop an informal pedagogy by, for example, offering tips and hints to writers or artists or using "beta readers" to comment on work as it develops. Such online practices challenge existing power relations between media producers and consumers and hold out the possibility of "a more democratic, responsive and diverse style of popular culture"—though the political consequences of such activity should not be overstated (Jenkins, 2003).

CONCLUSION: IMPLICATIONS FOR YOUNG PEOPLE'S MEDIA RIGHTS

The developments described in this chapter almost certainly necessitate a broader rethinking of cultural and educational policy. The traditional protectionist stance is no longer either desirable or realistic; however, it may be equally ineffective to adopt a liberationist approach, which simply asserts young people's freedom to choose. There is a need for "privatized" solutions that place a certain amount of responsibility in the hands of young people themselves, but there is also a need for more explicitly political responses in the activities of social and cultural institutions.

The notion of children's rights offers a useful reference point for thinking through some of these issues. The United Nations Convention on the Rights of the Child provides a number of general indicators: article 13 asserts children's right to freedom of expression; article 17 proclaims their rights of access to a range of media; and article 31 identifies broader rights to leisure and to participation in cultural life. However, like many such instruments, the Convention seems to leave it to parents or other adults to decide what is in the best interests of children and young people.

A brief sketch of what the media rights of youth might involve is presented below in four subsections reflecting the three well-established categories of protection, provision and participation, as well as a fourth category—that of education.

Protection of young people's media rights

Certainly the most familiar assertion in the present context is that young people need to be protected from harm. Young people, like adults, should not be exposed to material they have not knowingly chosen to be exposed to, or that might prove "injurious to (their) well-being".[12] In many countries there are laws against child pornography, indecent displays, and incitement to racial hatred, as well as strict codes of practice concerning false claims in advertising, the invasion of privacy, and depictions of sex and violence.

Arguments about young people's vulnerability tend to be used as a justification for denying them access to knowledge and power. There is considerable room for debate about what should be regarded as "harmful" or "unsuitable". A more protectionist approach might well deny young people access to much of what they are exposed to in everyday life, whether through various media or within their own environment. New distribution technologies significantly undermine the possibility of regulation either by the Government or within the home. On both philosophical and pragmatic grounds, it may be necessary to work towards the development of a system that supports self-regulation by young people themselves.

The issues raised above are particularly complex in relation to the Internet. Again, the solution may not be stricter centralized control or a technical fix such as blocking software. Young people who are determined to find hard-core pornography or racist propaganda will be able to do so irrespective of whether technological constraints have been imposed. There is a need for the more effective provision of information-both negative (in the form of warnings) and positive (listings of valuable sites, for example). A sustained form of education is needed as well. Young people, like adults, need to be able to protect themselves on the Internet, and to be discriminating about the information they disclose, not least to commercial companies. They also need to learn to better evaluate the information they find. Traditional questions about the ownership and control of information, and about bias and persuasion, are just as relevant to these new media as to the more established traditional media.

Provision and young people's media rights

With the rapid technological and economic changes occurring in the media field, new questions have been raised about the adequacy of media provision for young people. The sheer quantity of broadcast material available — at least for those with access to cable or satellite services — has increased enormously. However, quantity does not necessarily imply quality or variety. Continued regulation of both public and commercial providers is needed to ensure the availability of an adequate range of material specifically designed for young people in all their diversity. There is an ongoing need to finance the production and distribution of material whose commercial potential may not be immediately apparent in order to encourage innovation and counterbalance the dominance of a few select producers in the world market. Material produced by young people themselves should also be financed and made available via these new channels.

Inequalities in media access have increased significantly with the trend towards broadcasting privatization. These inequalities are especially apparent in relation to media for which provision is wholly or largely subject to the market, including films, books, and now computers. It is vital to insist on universal access, and to ensure that programmes for young people are broadcast on free-to-air channels in regular slots when young people are available to watch them.

Schools, libraries and other State-funded cultural institutions are increasingly being called upon to provide access to new media at the neighbourhood and community levels. However, access is not only about the right technology and hardware; it is also about the cultural and educational capital needed to use it creatively and effectively. Investing in technology infrastructure development by wiring schools, for example, is a merely symbolic gesture if it is not accompanied by investments in specialist staff and in training.

Finally, much greater consideration must be given to young people's own perspectives. Arguments about their cultural and psychological needs are frequently used as a justification for protecting the vested interests of adults and as a defence against change. In broadcasting, as in other areas of cultural policy, a dialogue must be created in which young people's voices will be heard, and cultural producers must be made more accountable to the audiences they claim to serve.

Participation and young people's media rights

The focus has thus far been on young people's "passive" rights of adequate media protection and provision; attention now shifts to their "active" rights in relation to media participation. Two broad types of participation are relevant in the present context: participation in production itself and participation in the formation of media policy.

The proliferation of new means and channels of distribution offers significant opportunities for the democratization of media production. This is most obvious in relation to the Internet, though there is no reason why it should not also apply to cable and digital broadcasting. What is needed is a forced incentive that makes the granting of licences contingent upon providing public access to production. Past attempts at providing such access to young people tended to be somewhat tokenistic; however, there has been some notable recent progress in this area with the distribution of excellent, innovative material produced by young people.[13]

Production opportunities for young people in other media will need to be made available in different ways. Media corporations could be encouraged, perhaps through offers of specific tax breaks, to sponsor and invest in community access facilities. In the light of prevailing inequalities in media access, such projects should be targeted primarily at low-income areas. Access to distribution channels such as community websites, publications and exhibition spaces should also be provided.

Participation also involves the assumption of a certain amount of responsibility and accountability for the functioning of media institutions. There have always been pressure groups that claim to speak on behalf of youth, but steps need to be taken to enable young people themselves to speak more directly and collectively to producers and policymakers. Regular regional conferences, preceded by web-based debates and linked to the media education curriculum of schools, would give young people an opportunity to make well-prepared contributions to the media policy debate on a more consistent basis. Likewise, resources could be made available for the creation of forums such as webzines or chat rooms on the Internet to facilitate dialogue between young people on critical policy issues.

Young people will only develop the competence to produce meaningful statements in the media, or to make their views known, if they are given sustained and well-supported opportunities to do so. Here, again, opportunities for participation need to be seen as part of a wider set of educational initiatives.

Education and young people's media rights

In the ICT/media realm, as in many other contexts, education is key. Educational institutions and providers—broadly defined—can play a vital role in equalizing young people's access both to media technologies and to the cultural capital needed to use them most productively. They can provide the means and the necessary support for the types of media participation identified above. They can also help young people develop the ability to protect themselves from—or more positively, to understand and to deal effectively with—the potential dangers of the broader media environment.

In many settings, media education has been relegated to the margins of formal education. It seems quite extraordinary that school curricula should continue to neglect the forms of culture and communication that have so thoroughly dominated the past several decades. A number of countries are working to develop or have already created a rigorous and coherent model of media education (Buckingham, 2003). A comprehensive media education is not confined to analysing the media or to some rationalistic notion of providing critical viewing skills; rather, it seeks to encourage young people's critical participation as cultural producers in their own right.

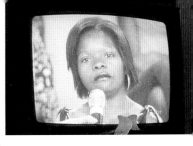

Media education is a very important dimension of contemporary citizenship-building and should therefore be seen as a basic entitlement for all school students. The nature and pace of technological change is such that different forms of media education that extend beyond the traditional classroom will become increasingly necessary. These will involve new types of dialogue between media producers, policymakers and young audiences. They may involve the creation of new public sphere institutions that provide all segments of the population with increased access to and opportunities for participation in the full range of old and new media. These and other such changes collectively represent a broader form of education about culture and communication than is currently envisaged by most educational policymakers.

Ultimately, media and cultural rights cannot be dissociated from the broader social and political status of young people. The call for cultural rights inevitably implies a call for political rights as well. In addressing the issues raised here within this wider context, important questions about power and access-about who owns the means of production, who has the right to speak, and whose voices can and should be heard-must remain at the top of the policy agenda. ●

[1] According to Giddens (1994), the past loses its power and influence as tradition grows thinner.

[2] Socialization is a concept that bridges the gap between sociology and psychology. Theories of socialization have focused on children's and young people's cognitive development (Piaget, Vygotsky), the psychodynamic development of personal identity in the structure of family relationships (Freud), the problem of social identity, the self concept (G.H. Mead), internalizing the group's moral values and categories (Durkheim) or perhaps multiple communicative interaction skills. Often a conceptual distinction is made between primary and secondary socialization, according to which primary socialization is limited mostly to childhood. Media in industrial and post-industrial societies is related to secondary socialization. (See Jary and Jary, 2000, p. 596).

[3] See, for example, Livingstone's perspective (Livingstone and Bovill, 1999); also see http://www.informatik.umu.se/nlrg/nlr.html (accessed 6 April 2004).

[4] The socializing influence of civic organizations did indeed begin much earlier, before the beginning of the twentieth century at least.

[5] This raises an interesting question concerning the quality of communal experiences on the Internet: Can there be peer groups without face to face interaction?

[6] See, for example, Stewart and LeSueur (1991) or the Online Journal of Space Communication (2002).

[7] See, for example, Parents, Media and Public Policy: A Kaiser Family Foundation Survey (Princeton Survey Research Associates, 2004).

[8] Some examples of these contemporary youth-orientated cartoons include Beavis and Butthead, South Park, Daria and The Simpsons, to name a few.

[9] The Columbine High School massacre occurred on 20 April 1999 at the Columbine High School in Colorado, United States. Two teenage students shot and killed twelve fellow students and a teacher before committing suicide.

[10] Dr. Francis B. Nyamnjoh, University of Botswana, as quoted in the report of the Fourth World Summit on Media for Children and Adolescents (Gigli, 2004).

[11] See, for example, the figures reported in "The youth vote" (Political Information and Monitoring Service of South Africa, 2004).

[12] Article 17 (e) of the United Nations Convention on the Rights of the Child.

[12] Some examples include Radio Arte in Mexico, an all-youth-produced bilingual community radio station that trains and encourages youth to develop self-expression through the broadcast medium (see http://radioarte.org); the South African show Youth Network Television (YNTV), created in 1995 by Ubuntu Television; Blast, a British Broadcasting Corporation initiative encouraging 13- to 19-year olds throughout the United Kingdom to get involved in media production, and Chat the Planet, a television show and Internet community that connects groups of young Americans aged 15 to 25 years with their peers around the world, via satellite, for honest dialogue (see http://www.chattheplanet.com).

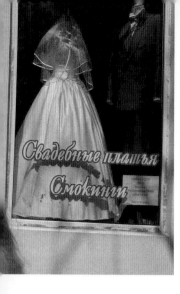

Bibliography

Abbott, C. (1998). Making connections: young people and the Internet. In *Digital Diversions: Youth Culture in the Age of Multimedia*, J. Sefton-Green, ed. London: University College London Press.

Barker, M., and J. Petley, eds. (2001). *Ill Effects: The Media/Violence Debate*. Second edition. London: Routledge.

Bennett, A. (2000). *Popular Music and Youth Culture: Music, Identity and Place*. Basingstoke: Palgrave Macmillan.

Brake, M. (1980). *The Sociology of Youth Culture and Youth Subcultures: Sex and Drugs and Rock'n' Roll?* London: Routledge & Kegan Paul.

Buckingham, D. (2000). *The Making of Citizens: Young People, News and Politics*. London: University College London Press.

_____ (2003). *Media Education: Literacy, Learning and Contemporary Culture*. Cambridge, United Kingdom: Polity Press.

Chandler, D., and D. Roberts-Young (1998). The construction of identity in the personal homepages of adolescents (available from http://www.aber.ac.uk/~dgc/strasbourg.html).

Curran, J. (2002). *Media and Power*. London: Routledge.

Cushion, S. (2004). Redefining youth citizenship: the Internet and anti-Iraq war protesters. Paper presented at the conference entitled Digital Generations: Children, Young People and New Media, London, 26-29 July.

Flench, C.E. (1999). Young adult authors on the Internet. *Book Report*, vol. 17, No. 4.

Frith, S. (1993). Youth/music/television. In *Sound and Vision: The Music Video Reader*, S. Frith, A. Goodwin and L. Grossberg, eds. London: Routledge.

Giddens, A. (1994). Living in a post-traditional society. In *Reflexive Modernization: Politics, Tradition and Aesthetics in the Modern Social Order*, Ulrich Beck, Anthony Giddens and Scott Lash, eds. Cambridge: Polity Press 1994.

Gigli, S. (2004). Children, youth and media around the world: an overview of trends & issues. Report of the Fourth World Summit on Media for Children and Adolescents, held in Rio de Janeiro, Brazil, in April 2004, prepared for the United Nations Children's Fund (available from http://www.ifcw.org/rio_research_paper_on_media.htm).

Hodkinson, P. (2003). "Net.Goth": Internet communication and (sub)cultural boundaries. In *The Post-Subcultures Reader*, David Muggleton and Rupert Weinzierl, eds. Oxford: Berg.

Holloway, S., and G. Valentine (2003). *Cyberkids: Children in the Information Age*. London: RoutledgeFalmer.

Jary, D., and J. Jary (2000). *Collins Dictionary of Sociology*. 3rd edition. Glasgow: Harper Collins Publishers.

Jenkins, H. (1992). *Textual Poachers: Television Fans and Participatory Culture*. New York: Routledge.

_____ (2003). *Interactive audiences? In Critical Readings: Media and Audiences*, V. Nightingale and K. Ross, eds. Maidenhead: Open University Press.

Kahn, R., and D. Kellner (2004). New media and Internet activism: from the "Battle of Seattle" to blogging. *New Media and Society*, vol. 6, No. 1, pp. 87-95.

Katz, J. (1993). The media's war on kids. *Rolling Stone*, vol. 130 (25 November), pp. 47-49.

_____ (1997). *Virtuous Reality: How America Surrendered Discussion of Moral Values to Opportunists, Nitwits, and Blockheads like William Bennett*. New York: Random House.

Kinnunen, T. (2003). *If I Can Find a Good Job after Graduation, I May Stay: Ulkomaalaisten tutkinto-opiskelijoiden integroituminen Suomeen* (The integration of foreign degree students into Finnish society). Kansainvälisen henkilövaihdon keskus CIMO (Finland's Centre for International Mobility) Occasional Paper No. 2b/2003.

Lægran, A. S. (2002). The petrol station and the Internet cafe: rural technospaces for youth. *Journal of Rural Studies*, vol. 18, No. 2 (April), pp. 157-168.

_____ (2003a). Connecting places: Internet cafes as technosocial spaces. Norwegian University of Science and Technology, STS Report No. 64-2003. Trondheim: Centre for Technology and Society/Department of Interdisciplinary Studies of Culture.

_____ (2003b). Escape vehicles? The Internet and the automobile in a global/local intersection. In *How Users Matter: The Co-Construction of Technology and the User*, Nelly Oudshoorn and Trevor Pinch, eds. Cambridge, Massachusetts: MIT Press.

Leonard, M. (1998). Paper planes: travelling the new grrrl geographies. In *Cool Places: Geographies of Youth Cultures*, T. Skelton and G. Valentine, eds. London: Routledge.

Livingstone, S., and M. Bovill (1999). *Young People, New Media*. Report of the research project Canadian Young People and the Changing Media Environment. London: London School of Economics and Political Science.

Martin, B. (1981). *A Sociology of Contemporary Cultural Change*. Oxford: Basil Blackwell.

Mead, M. (1970). *Culture and Commitment: A Study of the Generation Gap*. New York: Natural History Press/Doubleday.

Media Awareness Network (2004). Young Canadians in a Wired World — phase II: focus group (key findings) (available from http://www.media-awareness.ca/english/special_initiatives/surveys/index.cfm; accessed 6 April 2004).

Montgomery, K. (1997). *Web of Deception: Threats to Children from Online Marketing*. Washington, D.C.: Center for Media Education.

Nayak, A. (2003). *Race, Place and Globalization: Youth Cultures in a Changing World*. Oxford: Berg.

Net-Life Research Group (2004) (available from http://www.informatik.umu.se/nlrg/nlr.html; accessed 6 April 2004).

Nixon, H. (1998). Fun and games are serious business. In *Digital Diversions: Youth Culture in the Age of Multimedia*, J. Sefton-Green, ed. London: University College London Press.

Online Journal of Space Communication (2002). Issue No. 5: Satellites Address the Digital Divide. Ohio State University/Institute for Telecommunications Studies (available from http://satjournal.tcom.ohiou.edu/issue5/main.html).

Oravec, J. A. (2003). Blending by blogging: weblogs in blended learning initiatives. *Journal of Educational Media*, vol. 28, Nos. 2-3, pp. 225-233.

Petrazzini, B. A. (1995). *The Political Economy of Telecommunications Reform in Developing Countries: Privatization and Liberalization in Comparative Perspective*. Westport, Connecticut: Praeger Publishers.

Political Information and Monitoring Service of South Africa (2004). The youth vote. The third in a series of *Elections Briefs* by PIMS-SA at Idasa (available from http://www.polity.org.za/pol/opinion/judith/?show=48156).

Postman, N. (1983). *The Disappearance of Childhood*. London: W.H. Allen.

Princeton Survey Research Associates (2004). *Parents, Media and Public Policy: A Kaiser Family Foundation Survey*. Washington, D.C. (available from http://www.kff.org/entmedia/entmedia092304pkg.cfm).

Robertson, R. (1994). Globalisation or glocalisation? *Journal of International Communication*, vol. 1, No. 1, pp. 33-52.

Rosen, M. (1997). Junk and other realities: the tough world of children's fiction. *English and Media Magazine*, vol. 37, pp. 4-6.

Seiter, E. (2004). The Internet playground. In *Toys, Games and Media*, J. Goldstein, D. Buckingham and G. Brougere, eds. Mahwah, New Jersey: Lawrence Erlbaum.

Sharkey, A. (2002). The diffusion of community: rural youth, media and cohesion. Paper prepared for the International Sociological Association (ISA) World Congress of Sociology, Brisbane, Australia, 7-13 July 2002.

Shuker, R. (2001). *Understanding Popular Music*. Second edition. London: Routledge.

Sinclair, J., E. Jacka and S. Cunningham, eds. (1996). *New Patterns in Global Television: Peripheral Vision.* Oxford, United Kingdom: Oxford University Press.

Sreberny-Mohammadi, A. (1996). Globalization, communication and transnational civil society: introduction. In *Globalization, Communication and Transnational Civil Society,* S. Braman and A. Sreberny-Mohammadi, eds. Cresskill, New Jersey: Hampton Press.

Stewart, K., and M. LeSueur (1991). *To See The World: The Global Dimension in International Direct Television Broadcasting By Satellite.* Dordrecht, The Netherlands: M. Nijhoff.

Tapscott, D. (1997). *Growing Up Digital: The Rise of the Net Generation.* New York: McGraw Hill.

Times Mirror Center for the People and the Press (1990). *The Age of Indifference: A Study of Young Americans and How They View the News.* Washington, D.C.

Tobin, J. (1998). An American otaku (or, a boy's virtual life on the net). In *Digital Diversions: Youth Culture in the Age of Multimedia,* J. Sefton-Green, ed. London: University College London Press.

Turkle, S. (1995). *Life on Screen: Identity in the Age of the Internet.* New York: Simon and Schuster.

Ulrich, J., and A. Harris, eds. (2003). *GenXegesis: Essays on Alternative Youth (Sub)Culture.* Madison: University of Wisconsin Press.

United Nations Development Programme (2001). *Human Development Report, 2001: Making New Technologies Work for Human Development.* New York: Oxford University Press.

Volkmer, I. (no date). International communication theory in transition: parameters of the new global public sphere. MIT Communications Forum (available from http://web.mit.edu/comm-forum/papers/volkmer.html).

Welling, S. (2003). Youth and new media: framing the conditions of a milieu-sensitive computer-supported youth work. Paper presented at the EMTEL Conference: New Media and Everyday Life in Europe, London, 23-26 April (available at http://www.lse.ac.uk/collections/EMTEL/Conference/papers/Welling.pdf; accessed 29 March 2004.

Wells, P. (2002). Tell me about your Id, when you was a kid, yah? Animation and children's television culture. In *Small Screens: Television for Children,* D. Buckingham, ed. London: Leicester University Press.

Ziehe, T. (1992). Cultural modernity and individualization. In *Moves in Modernity,* Johan Fornäs and Göran Bolin, eds. Stockholm: Almqvist and Wiksell International.

_____, and H. Stubenrauch (1982). *Plädoyer für ungewöhnliches Lernen: Ideen zur Jugendsituation.* Reinbek: Rowohlt.

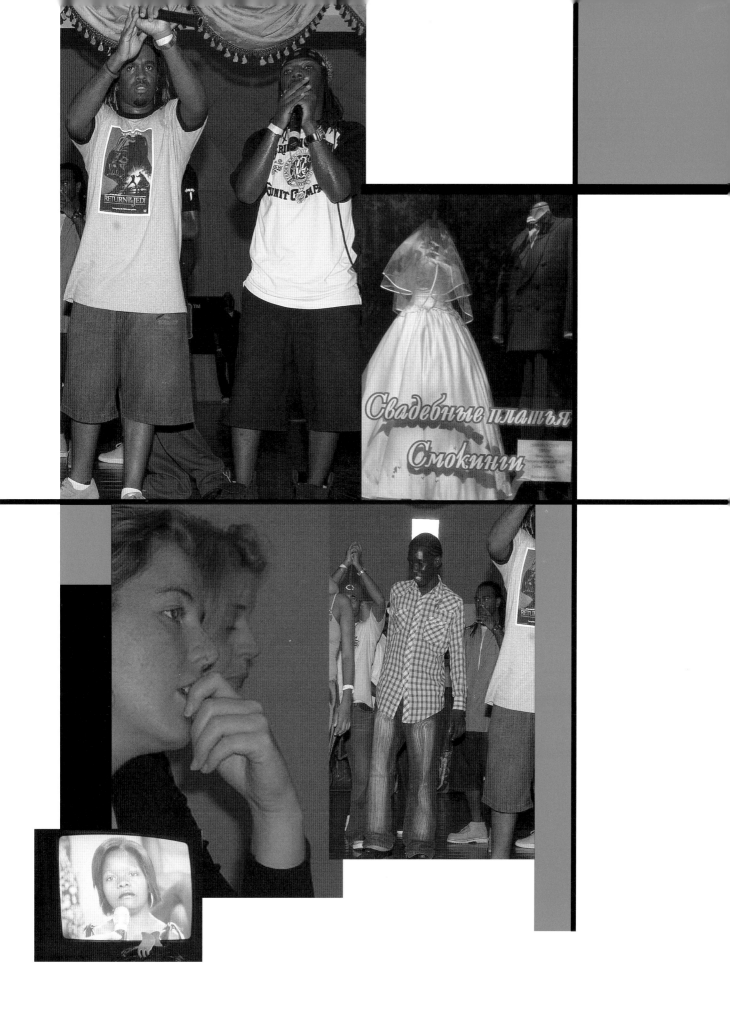

Chapter 6

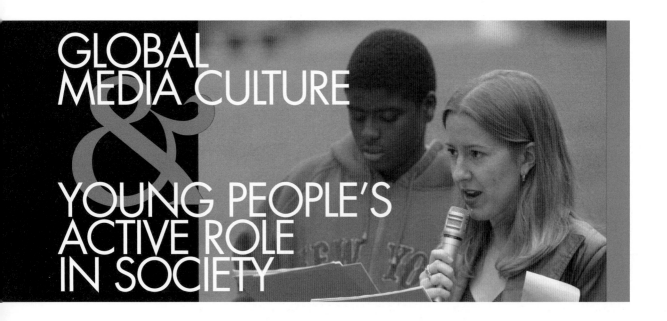

GLOBAL MEDIA CULTURE & YOUNG PEOPLE'S ACTIVE ROLE IN SOCIETY

The emergence of a global media-driven youth culture is affecting the way young people engage in active citizenship within their societies. Social and political activism is one of the means by which young people respond to change, though their participation in activism is far from pervasive in demographic terms. For example, while televised coverage shows mostly young faces at anti-globalization protests, it is clear that most young people do not participate in such demonstrations. Nonetheless, there is some evidence suggesting that more young people around the world are aware of and engaged in global or transnational issues than in the past; that ICT and youth-oriented media have both facilitated this awareness and engagement and helped enable an expansion of the types of socially and politically oriented activities that are considered "activist" by young people, which include but are not defined by participation in protest events; and that ICT is part of a new culture of engagement in activism that may have particular appeal to youth.

This chapter examines how the global media-driven youth culture is changing the lives of young people as active citizens and becoming a core component of their activism. An overview of young people as political actors is followed by an explanation of what constitutes activism (and what distinguishes it from other forms of civic engagement) and a description of the various kinds of transnational activism in which some young people are engaged. The chapter then highlights the ways in which technology and media are used by young people in various forms of activism, and how media itself becomes an object of youth activist concern. This is presented principally in terms of how young people are represented in mediated public spheres and how they can gain access to these spheres in order to speak for themselves.[1]

YOUNG PEOPLE AS POLITICAL ACTORS

The concerns that arise in societies with regard to young people as political actors generally relate to the kinds of citizens young people are right now, the kinds of citizens they will become in the future, and the kinds of things that need to be done to prepare them to become "good" citizens someday. Young people receive this kind of attention in part because they are presumed to be "incomplete" and not yet capable of fully responsible action and rational judgement. These concerns extend beyond the dividing line between the legal ages of minority and majority, which may vary within and between societies depending on whether the arena is voting, compulsory schooling, culpability for and jurisdiction over criminal acts, or overall personal responsibility and accountability. Even when young people reach a legally established age of majority, their formation as political actors is often regarded as incomplete unless and until they assume the normative status of an adult citizen by, for example, establishing an independent family household and maintaining full-time employment. The boundaries defining childhood, youth and adulthood may also vary greatly according to the context. In South Africa, the Youth Care Act defines a child as a male or female aged 0 to 18 years, while the National Youth Policy targets individuals between the ages of 14 and 35 to ensure that adequate support is provided for those who may face challenges and threats unique to this particular social group (South Africa, 1997). According to a recent survey in the United States, most Americans believe

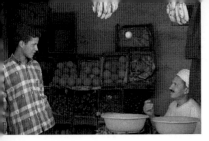

that grown-up status is not achieved until the age of 26, on average, and they see the attributes of education, employment, financial autonomy and family formation as key to being fully adult (*Reuters*, 2003). In Thailand, the Juvenile and Family Procedures Act defines youth as individuals between the ages of 14 and 18, while the Youth Development Plan identifies those aged 15-25 years as young people (Suktawee and Madkhao, no date).

There is a fair amount of research on young people as political actors; some work has concentrated on the present, some on the future, and some on the relationship between the two.[2] In Western countries, attention has principally been focused on voting behaviour, volunteerism, and the sources and effects of political socialization, especially civic education in schools. Much less is known about young people's participation in social movements and other efforts to change the policies or behaviour of powerful institutions. The study of social movements took off at the height of young people's political mobilization in the 1960s, which was characterized by anti-war, civil rights and anti-capitalist activism in the developed world, and anti-colonial, nationalist and anti-capitalist protests in the developing world. However, social science research on political activism in general and on young people's politics and civic engagement has tended to move along parallel rather than intersecting tracks. It should be noted that activism that is more publicly demonstrative and sometimes of a violent nature tends to gain far more attention than youth participation in non-violent movements or other forms of public advocacy.[3]

The activities and problems of young people have become popular subjects in a number of contexts, including social policy, public discourse and the media, and in line with this trend have also been subject to increased scholarly attention and analysis. These developments make sense from a demographic perspective, as youth have come to constitute an increasingly large proportion of the overall population in many developing countries, while they comprise a declining share of the total in many industrialized nations. In the developing world, many policymakers have been compelled by the growing "youthfulness" of their societies to place young people at the centre of the policy agenda.[4] In areas in which the age pyramid is reversed, such as Western Europe, concerns about young people are linked to issues such as immigration, given the relative youth of so many migrants looking for, and only occasionally finding, employment. Certain iconic events and well-publicized trends have also fuelled interest in youth in different parts of the world, among them high school killings, suicide bombings, the use of child soldiers, and protests by young people opposing liberalization policies around the globe. Certain issues of real or perceived significance have tended to dominate public attention and discussion, including the disaffection of young people from mainstream democratic politics (as measured by low voter turnout in elections), youth unemployment and child labour abuses, youth gangs and criminality, drug use, crises in public education, child sexual abuse, and access to "adult" content on the Internet, to name just a few.

Research is still catching up with both the myths and the realities of the contemporary lives of young people and with the broader implications of their ideas and actions for their present and future status as citizens. For a generation or more, research on young people in general primarily comprised social or developmental psychology studies of adolescence as a stage in the life course, or studies on youth culture and subcultures. Research in these areas is currently being augmented by work on a range of other youth-related issues that, while certainly not absent in the past, have gained momentum as discrete fields of study and/or focal points for cross-disciplinary collaboration and debate. Many of these topics are related to "politics" in its various dimensions and manifestations, with broad areas of concentration including the effect of policies and political and legal institutions on young people's lives; the ways in which "youth" is defined and used as a topic or category in public and policy discourse; and the ideas, values and practices young people bring to the public sphere. Specific issues addressed within this context might include youth employment and working conditions; poverty and homelessness; young people's political, civil, and economic rights; or the plight of young soldiers taking part in civil conflicts throughout the world.

Four core approaches to the intersection of youth and politics are presented below as a prelude to the section on youth participation and activism. These approaches may be characterized by the different terms they use to refer to young people, namely "generations", "adolescents", "youth" and "children". In different ways, they each contribute to a better understanding of young people's political ideas and behaviour and various dimensions of their political discourse, in terms of both how these factors influence the political trajectories of communities and societies and how they are affected by social and economic structures, various political, legal and media institutions, and diverse cultural contexts.

Youth in generational terms

One of the principal approaches to youth and politics derives not from a concern with "youth" per se, but rather from "the problem of generations".[5] This area of focus took on a relatively short-lived sense of urgency in the wake of the student uprisings around the world in the late 1960s and the emergence of the notion of a generation gap. The "problem" of generations has also been invoked at times in connection with nationalist and radical movements in developing countries as a framework or reference point for analysing resistance to colonialism or tensions between older and younger generations in newly independent nations. Discussions of Generation X in the 1990s tended to associate younger generations with political apathy. This approach lends itself to the study of major events and large-scale social changes and revolutions in which cohorts of young people play an important part.

What are the essential components of the generational perspective, especially as it applies to youth? Broadly speaking, it tends to focus on large-scale historical changes in generational politics across time in which "age sets", or cohorts, are a key element in explaining political transformations and continuities (Braungart, 1993). This does not imply that members of a specific generation possess a single political orientation or that consensus reigns among members of an age cohort. What is important is the notion that coming of age in a particular historical context imprints unique political concerns on generational members, who then respond to these concerns in a variety of ways.

In practice, the young people who receive the most attention within the realm of generational politics tend to be public intellectuals or catalysts of social movements—those who enter the public sphere to voice their concerns and sometimes claim to represent "their" generation and its interests. Very often, these "youth" are "students" from middle- to upper-class backgrounds who have the requisite cultural capital and social network connections to enter the public sphere as generational spokespersons or activists.

Overall, the "problem" characterizing this perspective relates to the ways in which new generations contribute to the political reproduction or transformation of their societies and the conditions under which this takes place. There is some attention given in this context to the intergenerational and intragenerational differences in political and other values that contribute to the emergence of generational political responses and activities.

Youth in terms of adolescent political development

A second approach to youth and politics, applied much more widely than the generational perspective, relates to the political development of young people and the nature and extent of their civic and political engagement. One telltale feature of this approach—not surprising given its connection to developmental psychology—is the use of the word "adolescent" in reference to a specific developmental category.

It is difficult to make any generalizations about this approach, though some broad tendencies can be identified. As with the generational perspective, adolescent political development is concerned with political outcomes, though far greater emphasis is placed on the quality of specific kinds of political systems (especially democracies) than on dramatic changes in political systems themselves. A good deal of work in this area is motivated by concerns that the quality of democracy is suboptimal and that this has a great deal to do with the political socialization, orientation and practices of young people. Individual processes of development and identity formation throughout the life course are seen as key to understanding the qualities of political processes. Adolescence is identified as a discrete social category in this context, especially in developmental terms, as it is one of those critical stages in life during which key values and ideas are acquired, with far-reaching implications at both the individual and collective levels. With this approach, youth/adolescents are principally regarded as "adults in the making"; the emphasis is on "becoming" rather than "being". For the most part, the adolescent political development approach is concerned with the kinds of "political adults" and citizens young people will eventually become based on their values, knowledge and experiences. It is therefore often linked to public interventions designed to influence young people's political formation within formal educational institutions (through civic education) and outside of them (see Sherrod, Flanagan and Youniss, 2002).

An important "extended" application of this approach, relevant to the subject of activism, involves assessing the extent to which youthful political experiences might influence adult citizenship and political activity. Researchers have conducted longitudinal studies and collected life histories in order to construct political biographies of young people, and especially of young political activists, to provide a better understanding this process.[6]

In comparison with the generational approach, youth political development is less organized around particular events or the broad social contexts or conditions under which political development and socialization take place. While these factors are considered important, they are not given the same priority as the development of individual qualities through family relations, education, peer learning, and experience.

Social context is the point of origin for approaches concerned with youth identities and cultures, though there is much variation within this perspective in terms of which contexts are most relevant. Although some early work was done on transformations in the notion of childhood in Europe (Ariés, 1962), youth cultural studies took off in the 1970s with research conducted in the fields of sociology and anthropology. The initial focus of this work was very political in that efforts were made to understand how young people made sense of and acted in a world characterized by socio-economic inequalities and racial and gender biases, with much made of the constraints they faced in this context;[7] over time, however, this field of research has evolved in many different directions, with only a few areas of study explicitly concerned with youth politics. Nonetheless, most youth studies are now united by a broader definition of "politics" than that used in more mainstream approaches. There is significant emphasis on either resistance or acquiescence to power structures, manifested in a range of cultural expressions and practices—such as popular music, style, drugs and criminality—that may not be considered "political" in the traditional sense. The young people who tend to constitute the focus of this perspective, including ethnic and racial minorities, the working class, or girls and young women, are often marginalized and stigmatized within the public sphere and at the formal institutional level.

Certain dimensions of the youth studies approach distinguish it from other approaches. It challenges the definition of "youth" as a stage in life and the notion of young people as primarily "adults in the making"; the preference for the term "youth" rather than "adolescent" is to some extent an implied criticism of the tendency to focus on what youth may "become" rather than on what they may currently "be". "Adolescence" is also criticized as being a largely Western notion not applicable to other parts of the world. The youth studies perspective is less concerned than other perspectives with issues of political socialization, and tends not to focus as explicitly on young people's attitudes towards democracy or on their political practices (if defined as activity within or oriented towards formal political institutions).

Another important dimension of this perspective relates to the ways in which the State and other powerful institutions such as media, schools, social workers and commercial enterprises contribute to youth identity formation through their portrayal of young people as either social problems or apathetic consumers.[8] This process, apparent in a wide range of public discourses and social practices—including curricular content, juvenile justice systems, the development of government youth agencies and programmes, and media representations—is rightly seen as an inherently political one. However, the connection between these external sources of youth identity-shaping and young people's political ideas and actions is generally not pursued in this approach. Its most immediate reference point is the emphasis on young people's "agency" in the face of the structural constraints governing their lives.

"Agency" is perhaps the principal focus of the youth studies approach in its present form and applies to a wide range of social practices and contexts, especially in the area of cultural forms and expressions. As mentioned above, many of these forms and

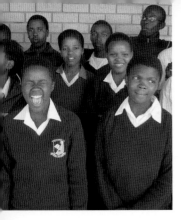

expressions are interpreted as having an inherently political content, particularly when they are seen to represent an implicit critique of or resistance to prevailing power structures. However, with the perspective currently under review, this kind of agency is rarely related to explicit engagements of young people in the public sphere through more conventionally defined political action or participation in social movements.

Youth in terms of children's rights, participation and citizenship

The fourth perspective on young people's politics relates to children's rights and citizenship. This is a more recent approach than the others—one that evolved directly from normative agendas and advocacy concerns (which are clearly present in, but do not constitute the central focus of, adolescent political development or youth studies).[9] The children's rights approach focuses on various local, national and international legal instruments and regimes as they apply to the lives of children and young people, their status as citizens, and their participatory practices in different arenas including local councils, national parliaments, schools, and social service agencies, with a lesser focus on their involvement in relatively autonomous peer groups and youth organizations.

This normative agenda, with its emphasis on the rights of children and young people-particularly their rights, interests and participation within a political context-both led to the development of, and is now inspired by, the United Nations Convention on the Rights of the Child.[10] The operative term within this perspective is thus "children" rather than youth, adolescent, or younger generation. The approach employs a legal definition of childhood (typically the period extending up to the age of 18) as its focus. This juridical differentiation between children/youth and adults is then used to argue for the need to "empower" children and young people in the political arena by both supporting protective legislation and promoting their participation; in the latter case, formal efforts might include lowering the voting age or guaranteeing young people's representation in public bodies, while more informal endeavours might involve facilitating different and more creative types of interaction (see van Bueren, forthcoming).

Like the adolescent political development approach, the children's rights approach focuses on young people's political participation. In the latter case, however, the key to such participation is generally viewed less in terms of political socialization than in terms of the rights young people possess or are entitled to. In this sense, the children's rights perspective is similar to the youth studies perspective in that both reject the idea that young people are adults-in-the-making and therefore not yet full citizens. It is unlike the youth studies approach, however, in that the identity of children and youth is seen as biologically defined rather than socially constructed, and the members of this group are seen to have their own sets of interests that require an enabling legal, political and cultural environment. The children's rights and youth studies approaches both place strong emphasis on the agency of young people, but in the former context this agency is regarded principally as potential or latent until an enabling environment is available, whereas in the latter context young people's agency is seen as an inherent part of their engagement with the social and political world.

Analysis of the four approaches

Careful consideration of each of the approaches outlined above contributes to a more comprehensive understanding of young people's politics. Two key lessons emerge from an overall assessment based on the application of these perspectives (which, it must be noted, serve as useful but individually incomplete analytical tools).

First, as is the case with other sources of social identity (including race, gender, social class and ethnicity), the category of "youth" is a heterogeneous one. Generalizations about young people are basically unwise given the diversity of their ideas and experiences across different geographical regions and within societies across the lines of class, education, gender, race and ethnicity. That said, special note should be taken of those instances — usually brief and episodic but often consequential and sometimes momentous — when significant numbers of young people develop and express a consciousness of themselves as "youth" and act upon this consciousness across various lines of division. This is where perspectives, approaches and examples relating to generational activism are especially helpful, both in understanding how this happens and why it is relatively rare. Media may certainly be critical in this context, as popular culture and ICT can serve as shared languages and channels of communication between members of an age cohort. As already mentioned in reference to bidirectional socialization, ICT represents an important aspect of the cultural differences between generations; its relevance in this context relates to the cognitive capacities and organizational strategies required for the use of media in political activism and other citizenship-related activity.

Second, young people are in a state of both "being" and "becoming". It is necessary to acknowledge their status as social and political actors in the present as well as their status as adults-in-the-making. The overwhelming tendency to view these two perspectives as dichotomous has limited research and activities in the field of youth and inhibited the development of new and productive ways of thinking about youth politics.[11] Cultural and developmental perspectives on youth have also been presented as either/or choices. On the one hand, a comparative perspective requires formal recognition and understanding of the ways in which the age groups identified as "youth" and the characteristics that divide this category from that of adulthood are socially constructed and vary from place to place. On the other hand, certain dimensions of age — including human capacities, the need for protection, legal and citizenship rights and responsibilities, and rites of passage — are ubiquitous. In other words, while the exact ages at which certain kinds of rights are extended, statuses are attained, and dependence and protection are superseded by autonomy will vary across time and space (and certainly between genders), these processes are universal.

It is worth examining how the media are perceived in relation to youth politics within the different approaches. Media receive by far the most attention in the youth studies approach, given its focus on both popular culture and the ways in which young people are publicly represented. Media, especially television, are also given consideration in developmental approaches, but largely as an obstacle to engagement and political development.[12] Until recently, generational approaches tended not to focus much on how the common experiences of an age cohort are shaped and shared (but see Edmunds and Turner, 2002). Clearly, wide use is made of the media in children's rights activism, but they do not constitute a central element of the analytical framework of this approach, which concentrates on legislation and empowerment.

One particularly relevant factor in assessing the role of the media in relation to local and transnational activism is whether young people are seen as citizens in the present or citizens-in-the-making. If the emphasis is on the latter, media may be considered instrumental in promoting habits that contribute to more responsible and informed citizenship (such as reading newspapers), but also somewhat problematic in that youth are seen as impressionable and easily manipulated. In this view, young people need to be protected from influences that might interfere with their formation as citizens. Society might even need to be protected from "misuses" of media by young people who are not completely aware of or responsible for their actions, or who show poor judgement (computer hacking is one example). Alternatively, approaches in which young people are perceived more as citizens in the present might focus on their ability to use media for activist purposes or, as will be explored later, as a distinctive means of engaging in activism. Regardless of which perspective is adopted, media education represents an important dimension of contemporary citizenship. It is critical that young people develop the ability to protect themselves from, or more positively, to understand and deal effectively with, the potential dangers of the broader media environment; it is equally important that they develop the capacity to take advantage of the growing opportunities within this environment.

LINKING THE GLOBAL MEDIA-DRIVEN CULTURE TO YOUTH PARTICIPATION AND ACTIVISM

Activism is a difficult term to define with any precision, as it is used in many different ways by a wide range of political actors as well as by practitioners concerned with the civic engagement of others. It is important to emphasize the "active" aspect of this concept in its application to young people's politics. For the purposes of this chapter, a working definition of activism is participation in any or all of the following:

- Protest events and direct actions (violent or non-violent);

- Ongoing advocacy campaigns to change the policies and behaviour of powerful institutions, including Governments, transnational corporations and international institutions;

- Consumer boycotts and other uses of market power to effect change;

- Information gathering and dissemination intended to attract media attention and raise the public consciousness with regard to issues of concern.

As suggested by this definition, activism is just one form of youth participation or civic engagement—and not one that is particularly common in relative terms. Other activities relating to youth politics and citizenship, such as voting, civic education, participation in debate clubs and informal discussion among peers, voluntary work, and service provision, may go together with or lead to activism, but quite often do not. Activism implies action that reflects expressions of dissent, attempts to effect change, or efforts to place issues on the political agenda. The definition applied in the present context is similar to

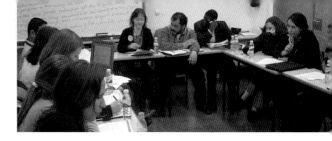

that used by Oxfam's International Youth Parliament in its recent report, which states that activism "can be broadly defined as efforts to create changes in the behaviour of institutions or organizations through action strategies such as lobbying, advocacy, negotiation, protest, campaigning and raising awareness" (Koffel, 2003).

The approaches outlined in the previous section reflect very different perspectives with regard to youth activism. The definition of youth activism used here is perhaps most consistent with the generational approach, given its focus on events and social movements. Adolescent political development would likely place these kinds of activities under the broader heading of civic engagement, but they are less central to its core concerns. Activism also plays a role in the children's rights approach, most directly in promoting the rights themselves. This category of political activity among young people may be of some interest in the youth studies approach, largely from the perspective of the cultural symbols and discourses deployed for political purposes.

As mentioned above, activism is not particularly widespread among young people (or the rest of the population)—at least most of the time. Even in comparison with voting, which typically draws a smaller percentage of youth than other age groups, activism is a relatively rare phenomenon. However, its importance cannot be measured by participation rates alone. The major protests and demonstrations that have taken place, including those connected with the "anti-globalization" movement in recent years, offer clear evidence that activism has an impact, even if the results are not always those for which the activists might hope. Activism may also have peer effects; even if it does not bring in new supporters for a particular cause, it is likely to raise young people's awareness of issues and expand their perceptions of what may be achieved through political participation.

One other issue worth considering is whether activism is, by definition, a good thing for the individual and for society. It may be virtually impossible to answer this question in the abstract; views will vary depending on the extent to which people's political goals and ideologies coincide with the objectives and activities of particular groups of activists. Activism must encompass a broad range of normative or ideological orientations if it is to be a useful concept for understanding young people's politics. From this perspective, youth activism covers right-wing anti-immigrant skinhead movements as well as anti-sweatshop campaigns, and the aims and practices of religiously inspired extremist groups as well as the activities aimed at social change among the younger members of mainstream religious organizations. In a sense, youth activism comprises a complex array of institutions and activities that are part and parcel of a functioning civil society and that are representative of its complexities and contradictions (United Nations, 2001). The term "activism" has largely been appropriated by those with "progressive" agendas centred around human rights and social justice issues, and most of the kinds of transnational activism reviewed below fall within that rubric. However, it is important to remember that much "non-progressive" activism occurs among young people who feel marginalized or threatened and seek to change the policies and behaviour of powerful institutions, and that the media and ICT are clearly critical strategic components of their efforts (see, for example, Wright, 2004).

THE LINK BETWEEN TRANSNATIONAL
YOUTH CULTURE AND TRANSNATIONAL ACTIVISM

Transnational activism encompasses a wide range of internationally oriented and organized political activities and networks in which young people may be involved. While there are no relevant detailed data with which to compare developments over time, it is likely that transnational activism, and especially young people's involvement in it, has grown dramatically in recent years.[13] There are several different forms transnational activism can take.

On one level, transnational activism may centre around issues or events that are outside the native country of the activist (an example being the human rights situation in another country), or that are global in scope (the implementation or strengthening of internationally recognized child labour laws is one example). Such activity might involve students from one country protesting against sweatshops in another country or refusing to buy the products of companies using sweatshop labour.

A second area of transnational activism encompasses the efforts of local activists to address problems originating from or caused by (or perceived as having originated from or having been caused by) forces outside their own countries. An example might be a Latin American youth taking part in an organization promoting debt relief or fair trade, or a Nigerian youth protesting the environmental practices of a transnational oil company.

A third aspect of transnational activism relates not to a specific issue, but to the networks and alliances that form between activists based in different parts of the world. Such arrangements may evolve in some instances, especially when the issue in question is considered global in scope, but not necessarily in others. This process requires a certain level of communication and even coordination across borders.[14]

There is a subset of issues in transnational activism with direct relevance to society's younger members; many young people engage in activism for the express purpose of improving their own lives and/or those of other youth. A range of global and transnational forces and institutions shape young people's livelihoods, life chances, transitions to adulthood, and effectiveness as citizens, either directly or through their impact on national and local policies and social outcomes; under certain circumstances these forces and institutions may become the focus of activism, including transnational youth activism. Activities in this area might include efforts aimed at halting the use of child soldiers or child labour, promoting youth employment creation, ensuring the extension of political and other rights to young people, protecting the legal status of youth in relation to juvenile justice and incarceration, reversing practices seen as discriminatory to young people (particularly when gender or race is also a factor), and providing wider access to education or health care.

Central to transnational activism is the linking of issues to particular institutions seen as being responsible for local or global problems or as having failed to address these problems. Media images of what has been dubbed the anti-globalization movement often portray various groups and their alliances as incoherent, at best, or nihilist, at worst, but in truth, most have quite explicit targets and audiences whose practices or opinions they want to influence, with attention often focused on the following:

- Transnational corporations, targeted because of their labour practices, investment strategies that exacerbate inequalities, influence on trade policies, and lack of social responsibility;

- Powerful countries and regions, targeted for their trade policies and agricultural subsidies (free trade for others but protectionism at home), domination of global cultural product markets and, most recently, military action around the world;

- International financial institutions, targeted for their structural adjustment policies, support of free but not fair trade, tendency to push for reductions in social services, and lack of participation in agenda setting and decision-making;

- Intergovernmental organizations, NGOs and humanitarian agencies, targeted for setting agendas independently from the countries in which they operate, using resources inappropriately, and displacing public sector providers;

- The media, targeted for stereotyping young people as apathetic or obsessed with consumption or violence, and for limiting youth access as producers of media content.

Underlying much of young people's involvement in transnational activism is the question of institutional accountability. Powerful institutions — many of which, in a local or national context, are considered "external" or global — are seen as having enormous influence over people's lives and young people's futures. However, these institutions are not accountable to those whose lives they shape, in the sense that the classic mechanisms of representative democratic government are not applied in a manner that forces them to assume direct responsibility for their actions. Transnational corporations, formally accountable only to owners and shareholders, are seen as even more powerful in an era that venerates the market and private sector, particularly since their identity is no longer bound up with, or their practices regulated by, individual States. Many young people around the world perceive this as a trend that will only grow with time, and they are concerned about how the probable widening of the accountability gap might affect their future and that of other youth. Most of the young people involved in the so-called anti-globalization movement are not opposed to globalization per se. Rather, they appear to be promoting a more accountable globalization, acknowledging the benefits of world interconnectedness (including economic relations) but arguing that such benefits are unequally distributed and do not offset the high environmental and other societal costs.

Clearly, not all youth respond to such issues by engaging in activism or other kinds of civic activity. However, research on activist organizations, ICT and "political consumerism" indicates that those young people who do seek a way to voice their concerns tend to eschew formal political institutions such as parties in favour of the kinds of activities that fall under the rubric of activism. In many cases, the cynicism about formal institutions and politics is linked to an idealism that compels young people to address issues of social justice and accountability more directly.

Engagement in transnational activism may be examined and perhaps better understood in the light of young people's civic and political involvement at the local and national levels. The way young people make (or do not make) connections between local issues that concern them (such as poverty or prison reform at home) and international issues (such as poverty or juvenile justice worldwide) may be especially revealing. It would be interesting to explore whether active young people in different social categories tend to focus on national or transnational issues. Are university students more likely to address transnational concerns? Do "active" marginalized youth concentrate more on issues of local concern for which local solutions are pursued (even if global causes of local problems are apparent)? These are some key areas for future research.

It is essential to gain a better grasp of what motivates young people to participate in various kinds of political activity (including transnational activism) and of the conditions under which different kinds of activism emerge, because the issues that resonate so strongly with many young people — such as justice, accountability, war and peace — are not likely to go away. What opportunities must exist or be provided for young people, and by whom, to encourage different types of activism? How are young people affected by their participation in social movements and by the success or failure of those movements? Is there a generational component in the rejection of formal institutional structures in favour of more informal processes (and to what extent does technology contribute to reliance on the latter)? Finally, does youth activism represent an embrace of the activist past of the parents and grandparents of young people today, the move away from which might be seen to reflect the hypocrisy and/or complacency of those generations in the present?[15]

TRANSNATIONAL YOUTH ACTIVISM, THE MEDIA, AND INFORMATION AND COMMUNICATION TECHNOLOGY

The rise of transnational youth activism and the explosive proliferation of new ICT occurred simultaneously in the 1990s. The relationship between the two phenomena is not easy to define; however, with what is known about the respective connections between ICT and activism and between young people and new media (especially the Internet), it may be inferred that the availability of new media technologies has helped shape young people's activism at a general level and has influenced the multiple and diverse forms it has taken. ICT has been central to global activism, clear evidence of which may be found in the documented activity surrounding the "Battle of Seattle", World Social Forum meetings, and a range of other global protests.[16] That young people are early and competent adopters of ICT and thus more likely to incorporate new technologies into their political and cultural activities is considered conventional wisdom among some scholars, not to mention many companies seeking to market new media technologies (see Suoronta, 2004).

Youth activism and new media technologies intersect in a multitude of ways. ICT is used for communication and coordination within activist movements and also helps to foster a sense of (virtual) solidarity among individuals and groups with different agendas and motives. Contemporary media have also facilitated the development of shared reference points for the world's youth. Young activists often incorporate globally recognized images and symbols from popular culture and commercial capitalism into their activism as elements of political protest and satire, expressed through political theatre, art, music, or dress.

The media are themselves a strategic target and platform for young activists, as illustrated by the following:

- The mainstream media are monitored for misrepresentations of young people in general and of activists in particular.

- Activists use the media to gain exposure for their causes and shape public opinion on issues of concern.

- Media access is a political issue viewed in terms of rights or justice; young activists often demand universal access to media and the right to become involved as producers as well as consumers of content.

Transnational activism is not a new phenomenon; abolitionists mobilized networks across various countries and continents in their struggle against slavery well over 100 years ago, and transnational networking was critical to the anti-apartheid movement in the 1970s and 1980s (see Keck, Sikkink and Klotz, 1995). However, the nature of such activism has changed dramatically with the advances in ICT. Contemporary global activism is in many ways defined by two key factors. First, young people now have immediate access to timely information on issues, problems and crises all over the globe, including detailed explanations of underlying causes and analyses of possible implications. Radio, television and the Internet bring these issues to people in ways that often provoke a visceral response, and offer a vast array of potential causes to fight for and villains to fight against. Second, faxes, cell phones, and the Internet allow wider and more immediate communication among activists once they have committed themselves to a cause; protest events, advocacy campaigns and consumer boycotts can be more easily coordinated, and bonds of solidarity may be established between people who may never meet face to face.

An interesting chicken-and-egg question is whether young people are drawn to transnational activism because of the use of ICT and the kinds of organizational forms that go with it or whether transnational activism is more high-tech because young people motivated to become involved for other reasons have pursued new media options to promote their causes. Whatever the case, the evidence is quite clear that those young people involved in transnational activism deploy ICT frequently and often effectively. Since the 1990s, in a range of protest activities centred around world trade and the global economy, "global justice activists have employed computer networks to organize direct actions, share information and resources, and coordinate campaigns through communication at-a-distance in real-time" (Juris, 2004). Mailing list servers, temporary and long-term websites, collective online writing and editing of documents, and online petitions are common features of transnational activism (Juris, 2004). Blogging has become a valuable mechanism for "technoactivists favouring not only democratic self-expression and networking, but also global media critique and journalistic sociopolitical intervention" (Kahn and Kellner, 2004). Even more individualized forms of political protest, such as decisions to boycott the products of a particular company, can occasionally assume a more collective character; for

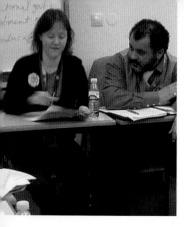

example, ICT can be used for "culture jamming", in which the public image of companies and their websites are targeted through Internet-based forms of protest and petition (see Micheletti and Stolle, 2005). Whether or not the political focus of transnational activists is interpreted as "anti-globalization" (a label most participants would object to), it is clear that they are using the core components of the global technological infrastructure to challenge what they see as the injustices of the global system.

As touched upon earlier, popular culture and the familiar symbols associated with companies and other institutions viewed by activists as unaccountable provide a rich collection of images from which transnational activists draw, often in ways that are satirical and entertaining. The global pervasiveness of these symbols and images makes them instantly recognizable to target audiences, whether they are watching protests on television or visiting the websites of activist groups. Using sarcasm and other such devices, creative activists can manipulate symbols such as logos or trademarks in ways that call attention to the hypocrisy of the institutions that propagate them to reap profits and instil brand loyalty. An example of such activism is highlighted in the following:

> The Canadian anti-sweatshop network, Maquila Solidarity Network, even distributes a Sweatshop Fashion Show toolkit, which has been used by young people across the country to raise awareness about sweatshop abuses in a fun and educational way. ... These tools help young people plan alternative shows whose purpose is the creation of public spectacles by questioning the politics of fashion products. Because of their alternative nature, these activities are often picked up by the media in various countries. (Micheletti and Stolle, 2005)

Popular music associated with different youth subcultures, including punk and hip hop, has fans and producers all over the world and is sometimes mobilized for activist purposes (see Ginwright, 2005; and Quintero, 2005). Alternative rock, played over independent or pirate radio, was central to the youth revolt in several of the former socialist countries of Central and Eastern Europe.[17]

The protest tactics outlined above, which involve co-opting commercial symbols for rebellious purposes, may be seen as an inversion of the tendency of corporate capitalists to appropriate the symbols of rebellion (such as rock music) for commercial purposes.[18] Analysts exploring this phenomenon from another perspective might emphasize that the very need of activists to use these symbols shows how pervasive they are.

Not surprisingly, transnational activists have established alternative media forms and outlets such as the Independent Media Center network to promote their views and communicate outside the circles of mainstream institutions. Interestingly, the mainstream media are being increasingly monitored and evaluated by youth activists, who are paying close attention to the way young people, especially those from poor communities, are represented in newspapers, on television and online. Negative stereotypes of youth, once unchallenged, are now more likely to elicit responses from organizations such as the Youth Media Council in California, which in 2002 published a report entitled *Speaking for Ourselves: A Youth Assessment of Local News Coverage*. In assessing the work of this organization and similar youth groups that oppose what they regard as the tendency to portray poor and migrant youth as criminals, analysts found that the "larger reason that (youth media activists) fight for media justice ... is that they believe that social justice is impossible without it since in their view ... media representations set the terms and conditions for a larger set of social issues" (Klinenberg, forthcoming).

Youth activists regard access to media, in the sense of being able to produce media content for broader audiences, as a dimension of social justice. Many youth are not content to remain passive consumers (another stereotype of young people) and see media access as an end in itself as well as a precondition for improving the lives of young people in other ways (see Kinkade and Macy, 2003). Though hard evidence is still fairly sparse, it can be surmised that activists, and especially young activists, see political struggles and media issues as inseparable and intertwined.

CONCLUSION:
NEW FORMS OF YOUTH ACTIVISM

The information and observations presented in this chapter raise important questions about the precise nature of the relationship between the emergence of a global media culture and the new ways young people are engaging in activism. It has been argued that today's global activism "reflect(s) important degrees of organization via communication systems—as opposed to communication merely reflecting or amplifying political organization" (Bennett, 2003). There is much debate about whether this trend is positive or negative, whether it is a sign of the strength or weakness of activist communities, and whether it is likely to help or hinder organized activist groups in achieving their goals. These points of contention notwithstanding, most observers share the sense that something new and different is going on in the ways activists organize, especially transnationally, and that new media and ICT are enabling and perhaps encouraging and empowering contemporary activism—though it is not yet clear whether a radical transformation has taken place.

It is worthwhile to identify those features that purportedly make present-day transnational activism different, and to explore the reasons for the apparent affinity between the newer modes of activism and young people. Transnational activism has been characterized as operating primarily through networks and loose alliances, a departure from the top-down organizational structures typical of earlier political movements. Members of transnational activist groups seem to view the participatory, consensual form of interaction and decision-making as a virtuous end in itself, and it is also presumed (correctly or not) that internal democracy makes the achievement of the ultimate goal of social justice more likely and sustainable.

It has been suggested that the newer style of transnational activism is characterized by the following: "(1) building horizontal ties and connections among diverse, autonomous elements; (2) the free and open circulation of information; (3) collaboration through decentralized coordination and directly democratic decision-making; and (4) self-directed or self-managed networking" (Juris, 2004). ICT functions as both an enabler and a metaphor in this type of activism; the Open Source Initiative represents a model for sharing information and the tools to make it available, but there is also a creative and occasionally mischievous and illegal model of hacking in which ICT is used to advance the political agendas of "hacktivists".

It is useful to consider how the four principles or properties listed above might influence young people's interest or engagement in transnational activism. It is not hard to imagine why a preference for horizontal ties, decentralized coordination, and direct democracy (the first and third items) might be especially attractive to today's youth. It is widely recognized around the world that young people are frustrated with and alienated from formal, hierarchical institutions — not only those held directly responsible for injustices, but also those involved in political mobilization (parties and other such entities within civil society are often seen as overly bureaucratized and therefore not internally democratic themselves). A connection is often made between these perceptions and low voter turnout among young people in many democracies. Only a relatively small percentage of youth make the leap into activism, but among those who are so inclined, transnational activism represents an appealing option because it is organized and conducted in such a way that it offers greater potential for consensus on broad goals and specific actions without the need to enforce narrow orthodoxies or establish rigid sets of priorities. On a normative level, transnational activism is more open to participation in that most members feel they are part of the decision-making process. Strategically, it allows flexible responses (in interactive, non-hierarchical networks there is no head to cut off) and the opportunity to move from one group and cause to another. It would be interesting to investigate how these organizational forms and features might appeal to young people in the context of their ambiguous status as not-yet-full citizens. Do they allow types of participation, agency and self-efficacy not available through more formal institutions? Are the features and tendencies associated with transnational activism-the informal structure, the idealistic goals linked to issues of justice, the sometimes uncompromising stances and penchant for risk-taking, the space for shifting loyalties and easy entry into new groups (and the associated process of identity redefinition) — somehow connected with "youthfulness"?

Self-management and autonomy (the fourth item in the list of principles and properties) might also be seen as bound up with youth, as this is the stage at which individuals begin to challenge parental authority and assert their independence. With the wide variety of causes available and the broad range of practices that may be considered "activist", participants in transnational activism can be part of a broader movement without giving up their priorities or control of their agendas. Is young people's involvement in such activism, with the autonomy it offers and the peer relationships that develop within it, at all akin to what those in the youth studies field would call a youth "subculture" — in this case a political subculture oriented outward towards changing the world rather than providing a haven from it?

Lastly, the emphasis on free and open information in transnational activism may tie in with the ICT-related interests and competencies of many young people and with the idea that information (in its multiple and diverse forms) is a public good and should therefore be available to all — a view that may be inconsistent with the protection of intellectual property rights. Young activists and non-activists alike appear to value open access to information, as exemplified by the activities of the Open Source Initiative and the widespread (but often unauthorized) downloading of music files from the Internet. If young people possess a generational advantage in understanding and using ICT, then new forms of activism allow them not only to participate but to excel and assume leadership. If access

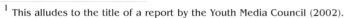

to information is highly valued among young people, they may be particularly motivated to develop creative networking strategies using ICT and are perhaps more likely to see both the production and the consumption of knowledge as part of the social justice agenda.

This conditional framing of the connections between youth, transnational activism, and new media and ICT has not been accidental. The understanding of this intersection and the accompanying dynamics lags woefully behind the reality of young people's use of media and ICT in the service of transnational activism. Even less clear is what kind effect all this will have on the civic and activist qualities of currently active youth later in life. What is evident from the involvement of youth in media-driven transnational activism — not as members of a "youth social movement" but as cross-generational partners with adults and sometimes leaders — is that at least some young people are asserting their (global) citizenship in the present not only by *becoming* but by actually *being* political actors. ●

[1] This alludes to the title of a report by the Youth Media Council (2002).

[2] For a useful overview of some of these issues, see Sherrod, Flanagan and Youniss (2002).

[3] For an exception, see Mische (1996). The involvement of South African youth in the anti-apartheid struggle, which fluctuated between violent and non-violent activity, is examined in Marks (2001). For an account of youth social protest in the former Yugoslavia focusing directly on media and popular culture, see Collin (2000).

[4] For a rich analysis, see Fussell and Greene (2002) and United Nations (2004).

[5] This phrase derives from the title of the influential essay by Karl Mannheim (1952), unquestionably the key reference in thinking about generational formation and its impact on political change.

[6] Perhaps best known here is Doug McAdam (1988); also see McAdam (1999).

[7] The still influential study is entitled *Learning to Labour: How Working Class Kids Get Working Class Jobs* (Willis, 1981).

[8] For an interesting discussion of these issues, see Mizen (2002).

[9] Indeed, for some in youth studies, children's rights advocacy has itself become an object of research (see, for example, Stephens, 1995).

[10] For an excellent analysis that finds mixed messages in the Convention on the Rights of the Child regarding rights to participation, see Lee (1999).

[11] For a recent discussion from the perspective of political philosophy, see Arneil (2002).

[12] For an overview, see McLeod (2000). The virtual demonizing of the effect of television is noted in Putnam (2000).

[13] The number of academic publications, journalistic accounts, and participant treatises and memoirs regarding mobilization related to global issues has grown voluminous over the past five years and shows no signs of abating. One of the few accounts focusing directly on young people's involvement is "Youth activism and global engagement" (Aaron, no date); also see "Using and disputing privilege: U.S. youth and Palestinians wielding "international privilege" to end the Israeli-Palestinian conflict nonviolently" (Pollock, in preparation). Youth activists in the United States have themselves recently published *Future 500: Youth Organizing and Activism in the United States* (Kim and others, 2002).

[14] See the influential book by Margaret E. Keck and Kathryn Sikkink entitled *Activists Beyond Borders: Advocacy Networks in International Politics* (1998).

[15] Recently examined in the United States context in Lassiter (2004).

[16] For recent overviews, see Surman and Reilly (2003) and McCaughey and Ayers (2003).

[17] For Serbia, see Collin (2002); for Mexico, see O'Connor (2003).

[18] See the subsection on changing economics in chapter 5 of the present publication

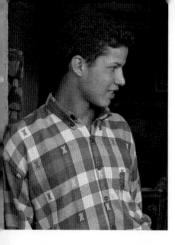

Bibliography

Aaron, P. G. (no date). *Youth activism and global engagement. OneWorld U.S. Special Report*. Washington, D.C.: Benton Foundation (available from http://www.benton.org/OneWorldUS/Aron/aron1.html).

Ariés, P. (1962). *Centuries of Childhood: A Social History of Family Life*. New York: Vintage Books.

Arneil, B. (2002). Becoming versus being: a critical analysis of the child in liberal theory. In *The Moral and Political Status of Children*, David Archard and Coin M. MacLeod, eds. Oxford: Oxford University Press.

Bennett, W. L. (2003). Communicating global activism: strengths and vulnerabilities of networked politics. Information, Communication & Society, vol. 6, No. 2, pp. 143-168.

Braungart, R. G. (1993). Historical generations and generation units: a global pattern of youth movements. In *Life Course and Generational Politics*, Richard G. Braungart and Margaret M. Braungart, eds. Lanham, Maryland: University Press of America.

Collin, M. (2001). *Guerilla Radio: Rock 'n' Roll Radio and Serbia's Underground Resistance*. New York: Thunder's Mouth Press/Nation Books.

Edmunds, J., and B. S. Turner, eds. (2002). *Generational Consciousness, Narrative, and Politics*. Lanham, Maryland: Rowman and Littlefield Publishers, Inc.

Fussell, M. E., and M. E. Greene (2002). Demographic trends affecting youth around the world. In *The World's Youth: Adolescence in Eight Regions of the Globe*, B. Bradford Brown, Reed W. Larson and T.S. Saraswathi, eds. Cambridge: Cambridge University Press.

Ginwright, S. (2005). Activism for the hip hop generation: urban youth and the struggle for social justice. In *Youth Activism—An International Encyclopedia*, Lonnie Sherrod and others, eds. Westport, Connecticut: Greenwood Publishing.

Juris, J. (2004). Networked social movements: global movements for global justice. In *The Network Society: A Cross-Cultural Perspective*, Manuel Castells, ed. London: Edward Elgar.

Kahn, R., and D. Kellner (2004). New media and Internet activism: from the "Battle of Seattle" to blogging. *New Media & Society*, vol. 6, No. 1, p. 91.

Keck, M. E., and K. Sikkink (1998). *Activists Beyond Borders: Advocacy Networks in International Politics*. Ithaca, New York: Cornell University Press.

Keck, M. E., K. Sikkink and A. Klotz (1995). *Norms in International Relations: The Struggle Against Apartheid*. Ithaca, New York: Cornell University Press.

Kim, J., and others (2002). *Future 500: Youth Organizing and Activism in the United States*. New Orleans: Subway & Elevated Press.

Kinkade, S., and C. Macy (2003). *What Works in Youth Media: Case Studies from Around the World*. Baltimore, Maryland: International Youth Foundation (available from http://www.iyfnet.org/uploads/WW%20-Youth%20Led%20Media.pdf).

Klinenberg, E. (forthcoming). *Youth Media Activism and the Decriminalization Question*.

Koffel, C. (2003). Globalisation of youth activism and human rights. In *Highly Affected, Rarely Considered: The International Youth Parliament Commission's Report on the Impacts of Globalisation on Young People*, James Arvanitakis, ed. Sydney: International Youth Parliament/Oxfam Community Aid Abroad (available from http://www.iyp.oxfam.org/campaign/youth_commission_report.asp).

Lassiter, M. (2004). Apathy, alienation and activism: American culture and the depoliticization of youth. Golden Apple Lecture, University of Michigan, 28 January 2004 (available from http:/www-personal.umich.edu/~mlassite/applelcture.html).

Lee, N. (1999). The challenge of childhood: distributions of childhood's ambiguity in adult institutions. *Childhood*, vol. 6, No. 4, pp. 455-474.

Mannheim, K. (1952). The problem of generations. In *Essays on the Sociology of Knowledge*, Paul Kecskemeti, ed. London: Routledge and Kegan Paul Ltd.

Marks, M. (2001). *Young Warriors: Youth Politics, Identity and Violence in South Africa*. Johannesburg: Witwatersrand University Press.

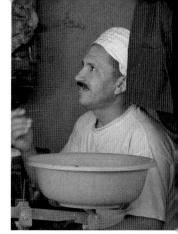

McAdam, D. (1988). *Freedom Summer*. New York: Oxford University Press.

_____ (1999). The biographical impact of activism. In *How Social Movements Matter*, Marco Giugni, Doug McAdam and Charles Tilly, eds. Minneapolis: University of Minnesota Press.

McCaughey, M., and M. D. Ayers, eds. (2003). *Cyberactivism: Online Activism in Theory and Practice*. New York: Routledge.

McLeod, J. M. (2000). Media and civic socialization of youth. *Journal of Adolescent Health*, vol. 1, No. 2, supplement (August), pp. 45-51.

Micheletti, M., and D. Stolle (2005). The concept of political consumerism. In *Youth Activism—An International Encyclopedia*, Lonnie Sherrod and others, eds. Westport, Connecticut: Greenwood Publishing.

Mische, A. (1996). Projecting democracy: the construction of citizenship across youth networks in Brazil. In *Citizenship, Identity and Social History*, Charles Tilly, ed. Cambridge: Cambridge University Press.

Mizen, P. (2002). Putting the politics back into youth studies: Keynesianism, monetarism and the changing state of youth. *Journal of Youth Studies*, vol. 5, No. 1 (March), pp. 5-20.

O'Connor, A. (2003). Punk subculture in Mexico and the anti-globalization movement: a report from the front. *New Political Science*, vol. 25, No. 1 (March), pp. 43-53.

Pollock, M. (in preparation). Using and disputing privilege: U.S. youth and Palestinians wielding "international privilege" to end the Israeli-Palestinian conflict nonviolently.

Putnam, R. D. (2000). *Bowling Alone: The Collapse and Revival of American Community*. New York: Touchstone.

Quintero, S. (2002). Black August continues: an exemplary blend of hip hop and political history for social justice. In *From ACT UP to the WTO: Urban Protest and Community Building in the Era of Globalization*, Benjamin Shepard and Ronald Hayduk, eds. London: Verso.

Reuters (2003). Are we grown up yet? U.S. study says not 'till age 26 (8 May).

Sherrod, L. R., C. Flanagan and J. Youniss (2002). Dimensions of citizenship and opportunities for youth development: the what, why, when, where and who of citizenship development. *Applied Developmental Science*, vol. 6, No. 4, pp. 264-272.

South Africa (1997). *National Youth Policy*. Pretoria: Government of the Republic of South Africa/Office of the Deputy President (available from http://www.polity.org.za/html/govdocs/policy/intro.html).

Stephens, S., ed. (1995). *Children and the Politics of Culture*. Princeton, New Jersey: Princeton University Press.

Suktawee, S., and M. Madkhao (no date). Thai definition of youth. Manila: Friedrich Ebert Stiftung Office in the Philippines (available from http://www.fes.org.ph/seayp_th.htm).

Suoronta, J. (2004). Youth and information and communication technologies. *World Youth Report, 2003: The Global Situation of Young People*. Sales No. E.03.IV.7.

Surman, M., and K. Reilly (2003). *Appropriating the Internet for Social Change: Towards the Strategic Use of Networked Technologies by Transnational Civil Society Organizations*. New York: Social Science Research Council (available from http://www.ssrc.org/programs/itic/civ_soc_report/).

United Nations (2001). *Report on the World Social Situation, 2001*. Sales No. E. 01.IV.5.

_____ (2004). *World Youth Report, 2003: The Global Situation of Young People*. Sales No. E.03.IV.7.

Van Bueren, G. (forthcoming). *Child Friendly Globalisation*.

Willis, P. (1981). *Learning to Labour: How Working Class Kids Get Working Class Jobs*. New York: Columbia University Press.

Wright, L. (2004). The terror web. *The New Yorker* (2 August), pp. 40-53.

Youth Media Council (2002). *Speaking for Ourselves: A Youth Assessment of Local News Coverage*, San Francisco: We Interrupt This Message (available from http://www.youthmediacouncil.org/pdfs/speaking.pdf).

YOUTH

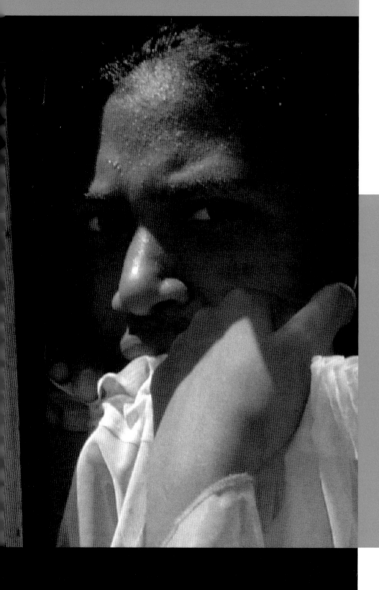

Risk

at

PART THREE

Chapter 7

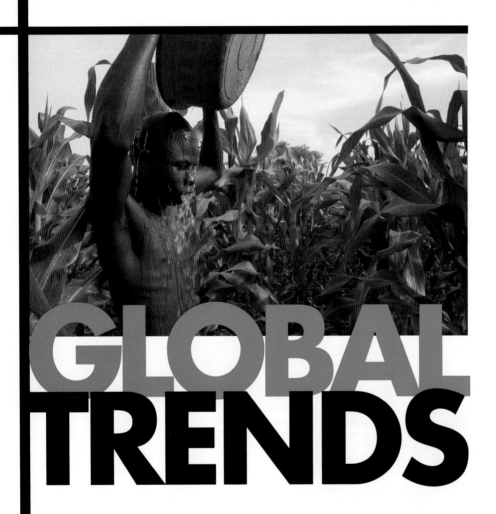

GLOBAL TRENDS

Most young people manage the transition from *protected childhood to independent adulthood quite well. With family, school and peer support, the majority of youth eventually find a meaningful place in society as young adults. A minority of young people deviate from this path; some engage in risky behaviour that can damage their social position or undermine their health. Many young people are beginning to explore their sexuality, and for some there are attendant risks. Some youth experiment with drugs or venture into delinquency, though such phases are generally temporary.*

These transitional risks have not changed much over the past several generations, and for most young people today they remain areas of primary concern. Since the adoption of the World Programme of Action for Youth to the Year 2000 and Beyond in 1995, the threat posed by the HIV/AIDS epidemic has received widespread attention. Almost 50 per cent of all new HIV infections are among young people (Joint United Nations Programme on HIV/AIDS, 2004). During the past several years, there has also been increased attention directed towards the situation of youth in armed conflict. A disproportionate number of young people, particularly adolescents, are involved in armed conflicts; they kill the most and are the most often killed. The attention of the international community has long been focused on the plight of child soldiers. A more recent concern is the emergence of "youth bulges"[1] and high unemployment levels among youth in various regions of the world, which could increase the risk of social strife and conflict.

Major developments relating to young people's health, vulnerability to HIV/AIDS, drug use and delinquent behaviour, as well as some issues of special relevance to young women and girls, will be reviewed below. In the context of examining health and gender issues in the cluster "youth at risk", it should be emphasized that gender equality and access to medical care and social services are basic human rights, and policies and programmes should be developed based on that assumption. Chapter 8 presents an in-depth analysis of the roles and situations of young people before, during and after periods of armed conflict, seen through a gender lens.

HEALTH

Health may be defined as a state of complete physical, mental and social well-being and not merely the absence of disease or infirmity. Because youth are a relatively healthy segment of the population, their health (with the exception of reproductive issues) has typically been given little attention. When they do suffer poor health, it is often a result of the effects of accidents, injuries caused by armed conflict, violence, substance abuse, HIV/AIDS and tuberculosis. Extreme poverty and undernutrition make some youth vulnerable to disease. Accidents and injuries are major causes of youth morbidity, mortality and disability.

Tobacco use is one of the chief preventable causes of death. There are an estimated 1 billion smokers in the world today, and by 2030, another 1 billion young adults will have started to smoke (Peto and Lopez, 2001). The highest rates of smoking among youth are in developing countries. Smokers are predominantly male, but the number of

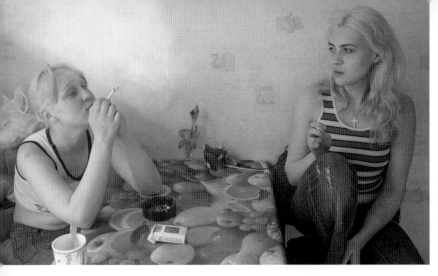

young women taking up cigarettes is growing. The higher level of tobacco use among girls suggests that there is a need for specific policies and programmes to counteract marketing strategies that target young women by associating tobacco use with independence, glamour and romance.

Despite efforts to restrict the advertising and marketing of alcohol and tobacco in industrialized countries, the youth market remains a major focus of the alcohol and tobacco industries. Some recent curbs on such marketing in developed countries have led these industries to concentrate increasingly on young people in developing and transition countries, where similar protective measures have not yet been implemented, and where, unfortunately, young people do not have access to the same levels of health and safety protection.

Young people worldwide are reaching puberty earlier and marrying later. Premarital sex is becoming more widespread. Despite a trend towards later marriage in much of the world, millions of girls are still expected to marry and begin childbearing in their teens, often before they are emotionally or physically ready. Data for the late 1990s show that among young women who were sexually active by the age of 20, 51 per cent in Africa and 45 per cent in Latin America and the Caribbean engaged in sexual activity prior to marriage; the corresponding proportions for males were 90 and 95 per cent respectively (United Nations Population Fund, 2004). In many developed countries, sexual activity is most often initiated prior to marriage for both men and women.

Many who become sexually active at an early age do not know how to protect themselves during sexual activity. Young women are often unable to negotiate condom use with male partners and may fear violence if they try to do so. One third—or more than 100 million—of the curable sexually transmitted infections (STIs) contracted each year are among women and men younger than 25 years of age. Having an untreated STI significantly increases the risk of HIV infection (United Nations Population Fund, 2004).

Although early pregnancy has declined in many countries, it remains a major concern, primarily because of the health risks for both mother and child, but also because of its impact on girls' education and life prospects. Births among women and girls under the age of 20 account for 17 per cent of all births in the least developed countries, which translates into 14 million births worldwide each year. In developing countries, one woman in three gives birth before the age of 20; in West Africa, 55 per cent of women do so. Pregnancy-related problems constitute a leading cause of death for young women aged 15 to 19 years, with complications from childbirth and unsafe abortion representing the major contributing factors (United Nations Population Fund, 2004).

During the past ten years, countries have made significant progress in addressing adolescent reproductive health issues, including the need for information, education and services that enable young people to prevent unwanted pregnancies and infection. Increasingly, these efforts are being undertaken as part of a wider, holistic approach aimed at reaching young people in diverse situations and equipping them with the skills they need to shape their own futures.

Drawing on the experience of the past ten years, a comprehensive approach to youth health programming has emerged as part of a global consensus on the need to link reproductive health interventions to efforts to provide adolescents with choices and options through investments in education, job training and citizenship development. It is imperative that health education, including the teaching of life skills, is introduced into both school curricula and programmes designed for out-of-school youth. Investing in young people's health, education and skill development, and empowering girls to stay in school, marry later and delay pregnancy are essential interventions that can substantially improve their chances of becoming well-informed, productive citizens. Youth health programmes and policies should be interdisciplinary in nature, extending beyond the health sector. Efforts need to be scaled up if the enormous health challenges facing the world's youth are to be adequately addressed.

Ensuring the full participation of youth in the development and promotion of health-related programmes and policies would enable them to become agents of change in their communities, improving their own lives and the lives of their peers. Youth who do not have a nurturing family environment, or who suffer abuse or neglect within the family setting, should be specially targeted.

Easy access to health information, general health services, and sexual and reproductive health services is a necessity for young people. It is important to ensure that health workers receive the training they need to provide youth-friendly services; they must be able to communicate effectively with young people and have the competence to handle their specific health concerns. Particular attention should be given to dealing with substance abuse among young people, immunization and nutrition, chronic conditions, trauma, and other health problems that may begin in youth but have implications for well-being in adulthood.

HIV/AIDS

The present generation of young people has not known a world without AIDS. As a group, they are especially vulnerable to HIV infection. Among the 10 million young people currently living with HIV/AIDS, 6.2 million are in sub-Saharan Africa and 2.2 million are in Asia. Nearly half of all new infections occur among individuals between the ages of 15 and 24 (Joint United Nations Programme on HIV/AIDS, 2004). Youth who are empowered to make informed choices have the potential and opportunity to drastically reduce the risk of infection.

Young people may be more likely than their elders to engage in risky behaviour, making them more susceptible to infection. A number of factors contribute to these circumstances, including a lack of information, peer pressure, an inability to calculate risk, impaired judgement because of intoxication, an inability to refuse unprotected sex, and the limited availability of, or access to, condoms.

The HIV incidence rate is higher among young women than among young men. One third of women infected with HIV are between the ages of 15 and 24 (UNAIDS Inter-Agency Task Team on Young People, 2004). The higher rates among women can be attributed to factors such as greater biological susceptibility, gender inequalities, sociocultural norms, financial insecurity, forced and early marriage, sexual abuse and the trafficking of

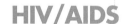

young women. In some countries, between 20 and 48 per cent of young women aged 10-25 years have experienced forced sex (Global Coalition on Women and AIDS, 2004). In sub-Saharan Africa and the Caribbean, young women are two to three times more likely than men to be infected with HIV. In Eastern Europe and Central Asia and in much of Latin America, however, young men are more likely to be infected than young women. In many regions, injecting drug users and men who have sex with men are particularly at risk.

The vulnerability of young people to HIV infection is highlighted by the fact that they constitute a significant percentage of high-risk groups in high-risk settings. For example, in several Asian countries, young people comprise over 60 per cent of sex workers, and in Central Asia and Eastern Europe, it is estimated that up to 25 per cent of those who inject drugs are below the age of 20 (UNAIDS Inter-Agency Task Team on Young People, 2004). In some regions, especially those with a high prevalence of injecting drug use, the age of initial drug use is declining. Young refugees and migrants constitute another group at high risk of HIV infection. The 120 million children who are not in school worldwide are also at a disadvantage, as they do not have the opportunity to learn about HIV and other reproductive health issues in a stable, credible classroom environment (Burns and others, 2004).

There are currently an estimated 15 million children below the age of 18 who have been orphaned as a result of AIDS, having lost one or both parents to the epidemic (Joint United Nations Programme on HIV/AIDS, 2004). Around 12 million of these children live in sub-Saharan Africa, and the number could rise to 18 million by 2010. With inadequate support systems and insufficient resources, they are at substantially higher risk of undernutrition, abuse, illness and HIV infection.

Intervention policies and programmes at the local and national levels should include life-skills-based HIV/AIDS education that empowers young people to make informed choices and decisions about their health. Young people will not benefit from the information, skills and services offered unless they are provided with a supportive environment within their families and communities and are safe from harm.

In order to reduce the vulnerability of young people to infection, steps must be taken to ensure the provision of high-quality primary health care (including sexual and reproductive health care) that is accessible, available and affordable. Ideally, health education programmes should be provided in this context, with particular attention given to HIV and other STIs. Community-based interventions have proven highly effective when specifically targeted at marginalized young people such as sex workers and injecting drug users, who have poor access to information and services and are at high risk of HIV/AIDS exposure. National policy should support these programmes and, at a broader level, ensure that an appropriate environment exists for reducing young people's vulnerability to HIV/AIDS and for implementing targeted interventions. Policies must be based on evidence of what is effective, and programmes should be scaled up in acknowledgement of the true scope of the problem. Continued international cooperation and collective global efforts are necessary for the containment of HIV/AIDS. Young people should be made aware of the full range of prevention options, with emphasis given not only to developing healthy lifestyles, but also to sexual health and behaviour issues. A behavioural change approach includes abstinence, delayed sexual debut, a reduction in the number of sexual partners, and correct and consistent condom use.

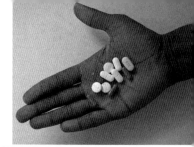

DRUG ABUSE

Adolescence is a period characterized by efforts to achieve independence from parents and other adults, by the formation of close friendships with peers, and by experimentation with a range of ideas, products and lifestyles. During this very fluid and sometimes volatile stage of their lives, young people often find themselves taking increased risks, making choices that may involve trade-offs, and taking advantage of opportunities that may lead to uncertain outcomes. The use of drugs, tobacco, and alcohol may become a means of escaping from situations that youth feel powerless to change.

Evidence suggests that young people in many countries are beginning to drink at earlier ages. Research in developed countries has found the early initiation of alcohol use to be associated with a greater likelihood of both alcohol dependence and alcohol-related injury later in life. Boys are more likely than girls to drink alcohol and tend to drink more heavily. However, in several European countries, levels of drinking among young women have started to match or even surpass those of young men. Data on alcohol use among young people in developing countries are relatively scarce, though some studies point to an increase in drinking in Latin American countries, especially among young women.

Growing alcohol and drug abuse in many countries has contributed to increases in both mortality and HIV infection rates among children and young people. In some Central Asian countries, the proportion of the population engaged in injecting drug use is estimated to be up to ten times that in many Western European countries. As mentioned previously, it is believed that up to a quarter of those who inject drugs in Central Asia and Eastern Europe are below the age of 20; further, the use of all types of drugs has increased significantly among young people across the region since the early 1990s (UNAIDS Inter-Agency Task Team on Young People, 2004).

Of all the illicit substances listed in international drug control treaties, cannabis is by far the most widely and most frequently used, especially among young people. However, what had long been a steady upward trend in cannabis use has levelled off in many countries in Europe over the past few years; in 2003, for the first time in a decade, there was actually a net decline in some of these countries. Data show that in a number of Asian countries, growing numbers of young women are using illicit drugs. Female injecting drug users are increasingly involved in sex work. In some Asian countries, the age of first drug use is declining.

A major development in the past decade has been the emergence of synthetic drugs. Despite efforts by many countries to limit the availability of amphetamine-type stimulants, a number of newer synthetic drugs in this category have become increasingly available. In most countries, stimulants such as methylenedioxymethamphetamine (Ecstasy) are consumed by young people in recreational settings such as rave parties or dance clubs. In developing countries, consumption is mainly associated with higher-income youth, while in developed countries consumption is spread across all socio-economic classes. There are indications that Ecstasy use is on the rise among young adults.

For programmes and policies to be credible and effective in preventing drug abuse, particularly long-term and high-risk consumption, attention must be given to the underlying factors that cause young people to abuse drugs.

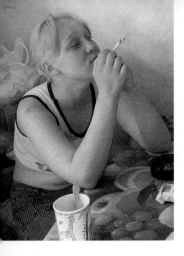

A more comprehensive approach to drug policy would include tighter restrictions on the marketing of tobacco and alcohol and greater emphasis on demand reduction efforts that appeal to youth. Demand reduction is a critical component in any drug control strategy, and national efforts should involve collaboration with young people and their communities in promoting healthy lifestyles and education.

Special strategies are needed for young people who are using or at high risk of using drugs, including youth from socially disadvantaged backgrounds, refugees and displaced persons, injecting drug users and sex workers. Initiatives undertaken to address drug use must constitute part of a country's overall strategy to reduce poverty, facilitate social inclusion, and ensure that the benefits of economic growth are accessible to all. Prevention and treatment interventions at the community level, combined with policies such as minimum drinking age laws and alcohol taxation, have proven effective in some countries.

Taxation may be an effective option, as young drinkers tend to have limited budgets, and their level of alcohol consumption is affected by price changes. In some developed countries, imposing higher alcohol taxes and instituting other preventive measures have been effective in reducing drinking and the potential harmful consequences of excessive alcohol consumption, including traffic casualties and violence.

JUVENILE DELINQUENCY

Juvenile delinquency covers a range of different violations of legal and social norms, ranging from minor offences to serious crimes. Quite often, youth take advantage of illegal opportunities and engage in crime, substance abuse and violent acts against others, especially their peers. Young people constitute one of the most criminally active segments of the population. Eventually, however, most youth desist from such activity, with few going on to develop criminal careers. Strong links have been found between youth victimization and the commission of crime. An overwhelming majority of those who participate in violence against young people are about the same age and sex as their victims; often the victims know their assailants (United Nations, 2005).

Young people who live in difficult circumstances are often at risk of delinquency. Poverty, family dysfunction, substance abuse and the death of family members are proven risk factors for becoming delinquent. Insecurity deriving from an unstable social environment increases vulnerability, and young people with poorly developed social skills are less able to protect themselves against the negative influences of a peer group.

Delinquency rates have risen dramatically in the transition countries; in many cases, juvenile crime levels have increased by more than 30 per cent since 1995. Juvenile delinquency is often highly correlated with alcohol and drug abuse. In Africa, delinquency appears to be linked primarily to hunger, poverty, undernutrition and unemployment.

Crime rates tend to be higher in urban areas than in rural areas, which may be attributable to differences in social control and social cohesion. Many of the urban poor live in slum and squatter settlements with overcrowded, unhealthy housing and a lack of basic services.

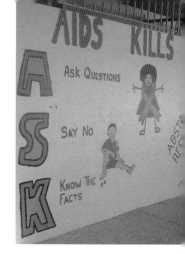

Delinquency is largely a group phenomenon; the majority of juvenile offences are committed by members of various types of delinquent groups. Even those juveniles who commit offences on their own are likely to be associated with groups. In some countries, youth gang activity rose in the 1990s as gang cultures were popularized through the media and as economic factors and a decline in economic opportunities led to an increase in poverty in urban areas. Involvement in delinquent groups works to determine the behaviour of members and cuts individuals off from conventional pursuits. The likelihood of experiencing violent victimization is much higher for gang members than for members of other peer groups. In one study, involvement in gang fights increased the likelihood of violent victimization more than threefold (Loeber, Kalb and Huizinga, 2001).

United Nations instruments largely reflect a preference for social rather than judicial approaches to dealing with young offenders. The United Nations Guidelines for the Prevention of Juvenile Delinquency (the Riyadh Guidelines) assert that the prevention of juvenile delinquency is an essential part of overall crime prevention in society, and the United Nations Standard Minimum Rules for the Administration of Juvenile Justice (the Beijing Rules) recommend instituting positive measures to strengthen the overall well-being of juveniles and reduce the need for State intervention. It is widely believed that early-phase intervention represents the best approach to preventing juvenile delinquency, and that the prevention of recurring crime is best achieved through restorative justice.

The policy options available to address juvenile delinquency and crime cover a wide spectrum but generally reflect one of two opposing perspectives that have emerged from the long-standing debate on whether it is better to "deter and incapacitate" or to "engage and rehabilitate" young offenders. The Beijing Rules state that "wherever possible, detention pending trial shall be replaced by alternative measures, such as close supervision, intensive care or placement within a family or in an educational setting or home" (United Nations, 1985). There is a danger of further criminal contamination when juveniles remain in detention pending trial, which argues for the development of new and innovative alternatives to pre-trial detention. Law enforcement is not the only answer to antisocial behaviour by young people, just as purely preventive or suppressive efforts are not very effective for youth already in contact with law enforcement. There is some evidence that community-based programmes are valuable alternatives to the locked detention of youth. It should be noted, however, that the detention of small groups of repeat offenders known to have committed the majority of registered offences does appear to have had a positive impact on crime rates..

Young delinquents often suffer social and economic exclusion. There is a strong reinforcing and reciprocal link between low crime rates and social inclusion and control. Over the past ten years, there has been a growing trend towards the adoption of effective practices that promote community safety and reduce crime in urban settings. Many of the relevant programmes are effectively targeted at the young people most at risk, or at those living in areas of high risk, and range from early childhood interventions, educational programmes, youth leadership initiatives, mediation efforts, and job and skills training to rehabilitation and reintegration programmes. To discourage violent behaviour and address delinquency, communities have to adopt strategies that combine prevention, intervention and other such options with suppression.

Though many changes have taken place in the composition and structure of families all over the world, the family remains the primary institution of socialization for youth and therefore continues to play an important role in the prevention of juvenile delinquency and youth crime. The most effective prevention efforts focus on the families of troubled youth, including young people with serious behaviour problems.

THE SITUATION OF GIRLS AND YOUNG WOMEN

Gender discrimination and stereotyping continue to interfere with the full development of girls and young women and their access to services. Education promotes gender equality in both the social and economic contexts, yet 65 million girls and young women remain out of school worldwide (United Nations Children's Fund, 2003). Five million women between the ages of 15 and 19 have abortions every year, and 40 per cent of them are performed under unsafe conditions (United Nations Population Fund, 1999). Studies researching young people's understanding of AIDS-related issues found that while both sexes were vastly uninformed, the level of unawareness was particularly high among girls aged 15 to 19 years. In almost all regions, young women fare worse than young men in indicators of labour market status.

Without gender parity in such key areas as education, health and employment, the goals of the World Programme of Action for Youth and the Millennium Declaration will not be achieved or sustained. Gender analysis and awareness must be incorporated into all strategies undertaken to address the priorities of the World Programme of Action for Youth.

Violence continues to be perpetrated against girls and young women worldwide. Physical and sexual abuse affect millions of girls and women but are seriously under-reported. In some African countries, well over half of all women and girls have undergone female genital mutilation; despite international efforts to halt this practice, its prevalence has not declined significantly. Women and girls comprise half of the world's refugees and in such circumstances are particularly vulnerable to sexual violence (United Nations, 2000).

Legislation is needed to protect girls and young women from all forms of violence. Particular attention should be given to measures aimed at preventing female infanticide and prenatal sex selection, genital mutilation, incest, sexual abuse, sexual exploitation, child prostitution and child pornography. There is a strong need for safe and confidential age-appropriate programmes as well as medical, social and psychological support services to assist girls who are subjected to violence.

Stereotyping and discrimination prevent girls and young women from participating fully in society, including civil society. Both traditional and web-based media continue to propagate stereotypes that often objectify young women and encourage restrictive ideas about their roles in society. Young people themselves must continue to be made aware of the harmful impact of gender barriers imposed by cultural beliefs, role perceptions and traditional practices so that they can practice equality. It is important that girls and young women have access to training, information and media material on social, cultural, economic and political issues and the means with which to articulate their views.

In 2003, more than 72 countries were identified as unstable (Joint United Nations Programme on HIV/AIDS, 2004), and 50 million people were living outside their communities or countries, displaced by conflict (United Nations, 2004a). A disproportionate number of young people are affected by armed conflict. They are most likely to be recruited as soldiers and constitute the majority in most armed forces, they are the primary targets of sexual violence and thus run a high risk of contracting STIs, and they are the most likely to miss out on education. In the past decade, an estimated two million children and youth have died in armed conflict, and five million have been disabled (United Nations, 2004b). Unfortunately, these individuals are the least likely to receive assistance (United Nations Children's Fund, 2005).

In environments that provide few viable options for employment, armed conflicts frequently offer young people a way of generating income. Providing youth with opportunities for meaningful work decreases the risk of their being recruited into or voluntarily joining hostile forces. In post-conflict situations, policies that emphasize strategies for youth employment not only help to provide a decent living for young people, but also discourage young soldiers from being re-recruited into armed conflicts. Special attention may be directed towards tailoring education, vocational training and skill development to the actual labour market needs of the areas to which young ex-soldiers will return. In this context, training has to go hand in hand with job creation in the formal and informal local labour markets. The success of such policies and programmes will depend on the wider economic and social environment of a country, including the trade situation, the availability of drugs and small arms, the extent of illicit weapons trafficking, and various gender-related factors.

The impact of armed conflict on the lives of young people and on society as a whole is enormous. Conflict seriously endangers the socialization process, affecting young people's chances of becoming economically and socially independent adults. Conflict often destroys the safe environment provided by a house, a family, adequate nutrition, schooling and employment. During conflict, youth health risks increase, especially for young women. Anxiety and depression, extreme stress, high-risk drug use and suicide are disturbing aspects of youth health that are particularly prevalent in countries experiencing war, occupation or sanctions. In the face of war and instability, adolescent engagement in risky sexual behaviour tends to increase. In countries in which HIV prevalence is high in peacetime, rates of HIV infection among both soldiers and civilians can jump dramatically during periods of conflict, spurred by an increase in sexual violence and prostitution, massive population displacements, and the breakdown of health systems (Joint United Nations Programme on HIV/AIDS, 2004). Trauma and the lack of social support and services seriously affect young people and cause lasting harm to their physical and mental health.

Over the past decade, a comprehensive legal framework has been developed for the protection of children. It is debatable whether this has contributed to a greater willingness among warring parties to look out for the needs of children. Experience from some countries in conflict does not indicate that achievements at the international political, legal and normative levels have translated into progress on the ground. Further, this legal framework is confined to children and young people under the age of 18 and does not apply to

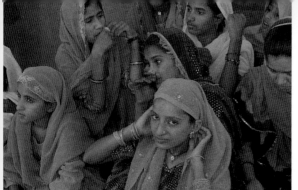

older youth.[2] In order to address the challenges faced by vulnerable young people during and after periods of armed conflict, international frameworks for action, including humanitarian and human rights laws and related guidelines, should be analysed and perhaps revised to ensure their specific application to youth in such circumstances. The rights and responsibilities of young people in and after armed conflict must be explicitly articulated in efforts to monitor, report on, and enforce international, national and regional commitments to youth. Work on behalf of children and adults must be more effectively linked in order to address the distinct concerns of young people.

In the context of young people and armed violence, the attention of policymakers and researchers is often focused on the involvement of large numbers of child soldiers in armed conflict and on the established link between youth bulges, youth unemployment and conflict eruption. While these issues are of great importance to young people and society as a whole, the excessive attention they receive means that the needs of the vast majority of young people who demonstrate constructive coping skills and do not become involved in the hostilities are often ignored. The diverse roles and experiences of youth during and after war, which go well beyond youth as perpetrators or victims of violence, must be further explored and addressed through diverse policy and programming approaches. It is essential to accumulate and exchange information on effective ways of responding to the special needs of youth both during armed conflict and after the hostilities have ended (during disarmament, demobilization and reintegration).

Youth should be engaged as central actors in identifying issues that concern them and in formulating solutions. The many initiatives of young peacebuilders around the world are evidence that youth are also agents of peace; with the right educational tools for crisis prevention and peacebuilding, they can develop the skills needed to help prevent violent and armed conflicts (United Nations, 2004a).

The *World Youth Report, 2003* provided an overview of the social, economic, political, health, psychological and cultural dimensions of conflict and their impact on the lives of young people, and mention was made of the frequent failure of preventive measures. The coming chapter builds on that overview, exploring the effects of armed violence on the lives of young people with the onset of conflict, during armed conflict, and in post-conflict situations, with a close look at gender norms and divides within this context. It also describes the gender gaps and achievements in humanitarian and post-conflict reconstruction efforts. The information and observations presented may contribute to future debates, as well as to policy formulation and programme design. ●

---

[1] Youth bulges occur when young people constitute at least 40 per cent of a country's population.

[2] The term "child", in connection with United Nations conventions relating to their legal protection, is generally used to describe all persons under the age of 18. The term "young adult soldiers" is used to describe individuals between the ages of 18 and 21.

Bibliography

Burns, A. A., and others (2004). *Reaching Out-of-School Youth with Reproductive Health and HIV/AIDS Information and Services*. Youth Issues Paper No. 4. Washington, D.C.: Family Health International/YouthNet Program.

Global Coalition on Women and AIDS (2004). Violence against women and AIDS. Geneva: Joint United Nations Programme on HIV/AIDS.

Joint United Nations Programme on HIV/AIDS (2004). *2004 Report on the Global AIDS Epidemic: 4th Global Report*. Geneva. UNAIDS/04.16E.

Loeber, R., L. Kalb and D. Huizinga (2001). Juvenile delinquency and serious injury victimization. *Juvenile Justice Bulletin* (August). Washington, D.C.: United States Department of Justice, Office of Justice Programs, Office of Juvenile Justice and Delinquency Prevention.

Peto, R., and A.D. Lopez (2001). Future worldwide health effects of current smoking patterns. In *Critical Issues in Global Health*, C.E. Koop, C.E. Pearson and M.R. Shwarz, eds. San Francisco: Jossey-Bass.

UNAIDS Inter-Agency Task Team on Young People (2004). *At the Crossroads: Accelerating Youth Access to HIV/AIDS Interventions*. New York: UNFPA.

United Nations (1985). United Nations Standard Minimum Rules for the Administration of Juvenile Justice (The Beijing Rules). A/RES/40/33. 29 November.

_____ (1990). United Nations Guidelines for the Prevention of Juvenile Delinquency (The Riyadh Guidelines). A/RES/45/112. 14 December.

_____ (2000). *The World's Women, 2000: Trends and Statistics*. Sales No. E.00.XVII.14.

_____ (2004a) Report of the Secretary-General to the Security Council on the protection of civilians in armed conflict. S/2004/431. 28 May.

_____ (2004b) *World Youth Report, 2003: The Global Situation of Young People*. Sales No. E.03.IV.7.

_____ (2005). Workshop paper 3: strategies and best practices for crime prevention, in particular in relation to urban areas and youth at risk. Background paper prepared for the Eleventh United Nations Congress on Crime Prevention and Criminal Justice. A/CONF.203/11.

United Nations Children's Fund (2003). *The State of the World's Children, 2004: Girls, Education and Development*. United Nations publication, Sales No. E.04.XX.1.

_____ (2005). Presentation on youth and conflict for the UNITAR/UNFPA workshop on population issues, 30-31 March. New York: United Nations Children's Fund, Adolescent Development and Participation Unit.

United Nations Population Fund (1999). *A Time Between — Health, Sexuality and Reproductive Rights of Young People*. United Nations publication, Sales No. E.99.III.H2.

_____ (2004). *State of World Population, 2004 — The Cairo Consensus at Ten: Population, Reproductive Health and the Global Effort to End Poverty*. United Nations publication, Sales No. E.04.III.H1.

Chapter 8

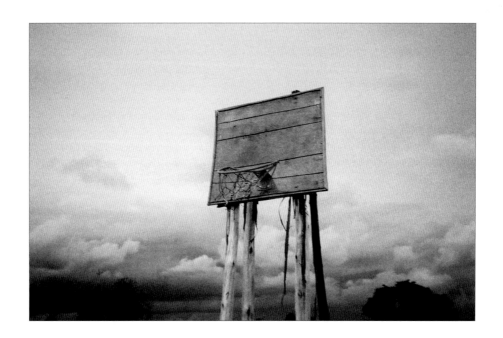

Gender dimensions
of youth
affected

by armed conflict

International interest in the situation of youth[1] affected
by armed conflict has increased in recent years alongside growing attention to the situation of children affected by armed conflict. The almost
universally ratified Convention on the Rights of the Child and its optional
protocols, as well as the reports on children and armed conflict prepared
by Graça Machel for the United Nations, have focused global attention on
children and war.[2] There have been a number of promising developments
in working with youth in conflict and post-conflict settings, ranging from
initiatives supporting youth civic participation and leadership to programmes addressing youth health, education and economic development.
Young people and those working on their behalf have urgently called for
more systematic and integrated support of youth rights and capacities,
including efforts to bridge major gender divides (including economic,
legal and social divides).[3]

While there is a vast array of child and youth experiences associated with armed conflict,
the direct involvement of children and adolescents in fighting forces as soldiers is the
issue that has captured world attention.[4] Global interest in understanding and curbing acts
of terrorism has also surged, and new research and policy developments relating to conflict prevention and youth reflect an increased focus on young males and their potential
for violence (United States Agency for International Development, 2004; Urdal, 2004;
Huntington, 1996). With attention primarily concentrated on these areas, the experiences
and capacities of the majority of other male and female youth who do not participate
in armed violence are marginalized, as are those of female youth who do participate in
armed conflict.

In international efforts to ensure that women's rights are recognized as human
rights, a significant amount of attention has been focused on the situation of women
affected by armed conflict. As emphasized at the Fourth World Conference on Women, held
in Beijing in 1995, armed conflict affects women and girls in particular "because of their
status and their sex" (United Nations, 1995). Systematic gender-based violence against
females in wars, including rape and other forms of sexual violence, is increasingly being
recognized as a weapon of war and a crime against humanity.[5] However, steps taken to
address these and other critical gender issues in conflict and post-conflict settings have
tended to enforce a hierarchy of gender action. Strong humanitarian programmes have
been implemented to assist girls and young women, but there remains a significant divide
between this work and work with women overall. Action in support of women often focuses
on those who have passed the stage of youth, not fully integrating the concerns of young
women and adolescent girls (Parker, Lozano and Messner, 1995).[6] In addition, limited
attention has been given to gender issues associated with males, including how they influence the critical gender concerns of females in and after armed conflict.[7]

As shown by the examples in box 8.1, youth and gender are both biological and
social factors that dramatically influence the lives of individuals and communities in situations of armed conflict. Youth have distinctive experiences of armed conflict because of
their age and their stage in life. These experiences are also strongly determined by gender,
or more precisely, by how the rights, roles, responsibilities and capabilities of females and
males are defined within a particular social context.[8]

Box 8.1

Some of us were traveling on donkeys [to the market]. ... Suddenly, the Janjaweed attacked us; they took our money and our donkeys. ... I was taken with my younger cousin to the wood. ... One of them forced me on the ground. ... They started raping me. I was bleeding heavily. ... It was so painful, but fear was even more than pain. Four of them raped me.[a]

— Nyala, a 16-year-old female internally displaced in South Darfur, Sudan, recounted February 2005

I went out with my mother to the market at Virunga to get some things. ... While we were shopping we saw a group of soldiers coming towards us. They told me to go with them. We knew they wanted to take me to go and train to fight. They took five of us-all young men-from the market. I didn't know the others.[b]

— Joseph, an 18-year-old male, in Goma, Democratic Republic of the Congo, December 2000

All day long, I move around in the city and collect paper-about 15 to 20 kilos per day. ... My father is disabled. ... Collecting garbage is a dangerous activity. We can get diseases. ... I was able to attend school for one year, but I had to stop for economic reasons.[c]

— Ahmad, a 15-year-old Afghan refugee in Peshawar, Pakistan, on his life as a "garbage picker", January 2002

"We have so many problems. ... We have no good shelter, no money; we are compelled to work. ... We will be beaten if we say no."[d]

— Fatima, a young Afghan refugee in Peshawar, Pakistan, describing her life as a carpet weaver, January 2002

Nyala and her cousin were targeted for sexual violence because of their age, ethnic background, and gender role as females; it was their responsibility to travel in and out of town to the market for their families, which made them especially vulnerable to attack. Rebels in the Democratic Republic of the Congo targeted Joseph and other young men for recruitment because they were male and of a certain age and physical maturity; they were believed to be able-bodied and, as males, presumably fit for taking on roles as fighters. Both Ahmad and Fatima are forced to work under hazardous conditions because of their ages and because their families must live clandestinely. As Afghan refugees living outside refugee camps in Pakistan, these young people are not officially recognized as refugees. Their parents have difficulty finding work, and both male and female Afghan youth in urban areas face major barriers to obtaining an education. As a result, an exploitative child and youth labour market flourishes. The types of work they do and the specific dangers they face are influenced by gender and cultural norms.

---

[a] Human Rights Watch, "Sexual violence and its consequences among displaced persons in Darfur and Chad", Human Rights Watch Briefing Paper (12 April 2005). A pseudonym is used for the purposes of this chapter only.

[b] Human Rights Watch, "Reluctant recruits: children and adults forcibly recruited for military service in North Kivu, Democratic Republic of the Congo", *Human Rights Watch*, vol. 13, No. 3A (May 2001). A pseudonym is used for the purposes of this chapter only.

[c] Jane Lowicki, *Fending for Themselves, Afghan Refugee Children and Adolescents Working in Urban Pakistan*, Women's Commission for Refugee Women and Children, Mission to Pakistan, January 2002 (New York: Women's Commission for Refugee Women and Children, May 2002), p. 11.

[d] Ibid., p. 9.

In spite of their combined relevance, youth and gender are rarely considered together in efforts to understand and address the dynamics of armed conflict. When these factors are assessed individually, attention is often narrowly focused on limited or stereotypical experiences of male and female youth. The consequent failure to recognize the complexity of issues facing youth affected by armed conflict results in the loss of opportunities to more effectively support the protection and development of young people and the overall well-being of their societies. As figure 8.1 shows, the simultaneous consideration of youth and gender requires attention to the age- and gender-specific experiences of both females and males in a given context.

Figure 8.1
Combined gender and youth analysis

		Youth analysis		
		Children	Youth	Adults
Gender analysis	Females			
	Males			

A combined and expanded gender and youth analysis requires looking at armed conflict from different perspectives in order to gain a better understanding of its complexity and the diversity of youth experiences in conflict situations. Among other things, applying a gender analysis should stimulate discussion and action in response to the many questions that are certain to emerge, particularly with regard to underlying factors and motivations. What drives young males to pick up weapons? What are the gender norms and values that enforce the roles of youth in this context and block access to social discourse and decision-making for females and males who seek non-violent paths to survival, conflict resolution and well-being? Gender analysis can better define the roles of both male and female youth in perpetuating armed conflict, and can reveal the ways in which armed conflict not only exacerbates gender inequalities, discrimination and abuse, but also challenges gender roles and presents opportunities for positive social change, with youth at the helm. Applying a youth analysis exposes the need to systematically support the rights of youth so that their distinct roles and capacities for survival, community recovery and conflict prevention are not sidestepped or subsumed under programmes for children or adults.

This chapter highlights some of the dynamics associated with youth and gender in armed conflict and post-conflict situations. Gender and youth as social constructs are defined in greater detail. A description of the key issues facing youth before, in and after conflict is provided, revealing tremendous abuses, social upheaval and other challenges experienced by young people as a consequence of their gender or stage in the life cycle. An analysis of achievements and gaps in addressing the gender- and age-related problems of young people affected by armed conflict is also provided, followed by a number of recommendations on ways to move forward, including suggestions on support for youth-informed and youth-driven solutions that take into account both youth- and gender-based concerns.

WHAT DOES "GENDER" MEAN? WHO ARE "YOUTH AFFECTED BY ARMED CONFLICT"?

What is gender, and why is it important to consider in relation to armed conflicts? What is unique about youth? What makes them different from older adults or younger children? Why do they require distinct attention in armed conflict and post-conflict situations?

Gender

Gender refers not only to the physiological or sex differences between females and males, but also to those that are socially constructed. Males and females are biologically different in many ways, primarily in terms of their reproductive functions, but they may also be differentiated by socially constructed beliefs about what it means to be male or female. The concept of gender applies to the relationships between females and males individually and within their societies and communities as they are socially defined. These relationships are characterized by differences in gender roles, the division of labour, power relations, and access to resources, information, decision-making processes, and other assets or benefits. While the biology, or sex, of females and males does not change across cultures, time or space, gender beliefs and relationships are constantly changing and may vary greatly between cultures and locales and over time. As indicated here, the term gender refers to much more than the physical differences between males and females.[9]

Gender norms and divides

Gender norms are created and perpetuated in every society based on a range of political, social, cultural, economic and other circumstances. These norms are not biologically mandated but instead represent social perceptions of masculinity and femininity and beliefs about the ways males and females should think, feel, act and interact. For example, though females may give birth, child-rearing does not inherently need to be carried out exclusively or predominantly by females or males. Some common gender-role stereotypes include females as caregivers, homemakers, nurturers, wives, mothers and victims; and males as protectors, providers, decision makers, heads of household and aggressors. Beliefs about the roles and capacities of females and males also shape the division of labour, defining "women's work" and "men's work". In societies with traditional gender-role expectations, females may be the water gatherers, market sellers, food preparers, nurses and teachers, while males may be the hunters, politicians, drivers, carpenters, doctors, soldiers, and members of the clergy.

While many males and females do take on these more stereotypical gender roles, in reality, males and females around the world do all of these things and play multiple and varied roles in their families, communities and societies depending on the specific context. Many females are soldiers, heads of household, and the sole income earners for their families. Many males are teachers, cooks and nurturers, and they may also be victimized, contrary to the stereotypical view of males as "aggressors". The inability to see beyond gender stereotypes and recognize the diversity of roles males and females play reinforces erroneous assumptions about their capacities and needs. This gender blindness directly affects how youth are supported in diverse and dynamic social and gender environments, including armed conflict and post-conflict settings (El-Jack, 2003).

Most characterizations of gender norms reflect those of adult women and men rather than those of children, adolescents or youth. Young people's gender roles are often defined in relation to adult roles. Vis-à-vis children and youth, adults typically perform the roles of parents, providers, protectors, teachers, authority figures and disciplinarians. Young people are often considered subordinate dependants, learners and helpers, carrying out or assisting with the gendered tasks expected of their sex as adults. For example, girls' roles may include gathering water, caring for younger children, cooking and serving food, and doing the washing up, either alongside or in place of their mothers or other elder females. Boys may be expected to join armies, defend their villages, or earn wages along with or in place of their fathers or other older men. In their own right, many youth also take on roles as parents, wives, husbands, students, workers, providers and more. As with adults, both male and female children and youth may do all of these things in a range of contexts.

For many, the behaviour of youth represents a strong indicator of the current and future well-being of families and entire communities. If some participate in violence or otherwise deviate from accepted social norms, it may cast all roles youth play in their society into a negative light.

Despite the diversity of female and male gender roles around the world, there are major gender divides at both the interpersonal and structural levels that are disproportionately devastating to females. As a result of gender inequalities involving unequal power relations between males and females, women and girls are often discriminated against and do not enjoy equal access to the means of securing or safeguarding their human rights. Relegated to a subordinate status, females are often denied basic rights to life, equality, security of the person, equal protection under the law, and freedom from torture and other cruel, inhumane or degrading treatment.

In societies controlled principally by men, females may not be allowed to inherit or own property; to make decisions freely, including those relating to marriage, divorce and their fertility; to secure employment, receive equal pay for equal work, and become self-sufficient; or to ensure that they are protected against sexual abuse and exploitation and other violence. As explained in greater detail below, females are the principal targets of gender-based violence, including rape and sexual assault. National laws and enforcement authorities may reinforce or even perpetuate gender-based violence and gender discrimination against females instead of providing them with protection.

Women and girls are, on the whole, far less likely than males to command resources, and they comprise the majority of the world's economically poor (United Nations, 1997; United Nations Development Programme, 2003; Coleman, 2005). As such, they are more vulnerable to contracting HIV as a result of sexual exploitation and abuse and poor health care, all of which are exacerbated by economic deprivation. Many females and males are uninformed about the rights of women and girls, and about human rights in general. Even when they are informed, legal support for challenging customary practices such as a "husband's right" to beat his wife is often not available. Females do not always have the resources to secure legal representation, let alone support systems that will help them deal with the wider social recriminations that accompany efforts to ensure the enforcement of their legal rights. Local cultural norms may also be held to supersede international norms, including by aid groups concerned about imposing culture.

Young women often face a double barrier to gender equality owing to their age and status in society. Not only are they abused and disadvantaged in the ways described, but they may have even less access to resources and support and be less able to assert their rights than older women. Although women's and children's rights have been articulated internationally, there has been a failure to ensure the explicit expression of youth rights on the same scale, as a result of which they may not receive the same level of recognition and support.

Gender divides may greatly affect males as well. As described later, males also experience gender-based violence, as they may be targets for murder, sexual violence and forced soldiering. Their overall well-being and that of their societies are affected by the lower economic and social status of their mothers and sisters, who play major caregiving and protective roles, often with little access to health care and other resources.

As noted later in the chapter, gender divides often worsen during and after armed conflicts, though such situations may also present opportunities for social transformation and improvements in gender equality.

Youth

Youth represents the transition from childhood to adulthood and is therefore a dynamic stage in an individual's development. It is an important period of physical, mental and social maturation, during which young people are actively forming their identities and determining acceptable roles for themselves within their communities and societies. They are increasingly capable of abstract thought and independent decision-making. As their bodies continue to change, their sexuality begins to emerge, and they are presented with new physical and emotional feelings as well as new social expectations and challenges.

Youth is often a period of risk-taking, when young people push boundaries and at times engage in conflict with adults and others as they seek to confirm or disprove what they feel they know about themselves, their world, and the limits of acceptable behaviour. Some youth may be extremely politically minded, concerned about social conditions, ideals-driven and action-oriented. Others, often especially female youth, are socialized to be silent and compliant as the greatest proof of their maturity and adulthood. Youth, ultimately, are seeking connection, care, the ability to care for themselves and others effectively, and a role and identity in society.

Most countries have a legally defined age of majority at which an individual assumes the full rights and responsibilities of an adult under the law. In most countries, the legal age of majority is 18, which is compatible with the definition of children as those between the ages of 0 and 18 in the almost universally ratified Convention on the Rights of the Child. United Nations agencies also employ various working definitions that apply to the period between childhood and adulthood: adolescents are defined as those aged 10 to 19 years; youth as those between the ages of 15 and 24; young people as those aged 10 to 24 years; and adults as those aged 18 years and above.[10] How young people view themselves and are viewed by their societies in day-to-day life is often very different, however.

Concepts surrounding the period and definition of youth vary greatly across societies and cultural contexts, including along gender lines. At times, youth over the age of 18 are not considered to be adults by their societies because they have not met other social criteria. For many girls in Sierra Leone, for example, the way to be accepted as a woman in society is to be inducted into a Secret Society and to have undergone female genital mutilation (FGM), making the woman eligible for marriage. By contrast, there are many young people under the age of 18 who are already seen as adults. In many parts of the world, 12- and 13-year-old girls are considered to be adult women when they marry, and this shift in status requires them to leave school and assume household responsibilities full-time. In the Xhosa tradition in South Africa, boys become men through circumcision. They participate in a lengthy and elaborate ritual in preparation for manhood, after which they are allowed to inherit, marry and officiate in tribal rituals (Mandela, 1994). These types of sociocultural transformations, or rites of passage, often involve the transfer of cultural and other learning, as well as resources, from adults to young people to ease their transition into parenting, earning a livelihood, or other aspects of adult functioning.

As these examples indicate, formal definitions of youth may be based on age, but the concept of youth is ultimately culturally and contextually bound by the customs and belief systems of societies and even individual families. In armed conflict, the social support systems and roles of children, youth and adults undergo tremendous, deliberate upheaval. Young people affected by armed conflict are often forced to take on new roles without full preparation, support or community sanction, at times modifying or transforming the adult and gender roles they have assumed. Those attempting to identify and work with youth affected by armed conflict must take into account the dynamic social changes under way and not simply rely on old norms in anticipating and devising solutions to address youth concerns (Lowicki-Zucca, 2004a; 2004b).

Youth affected by armed conflict

International and civil wars, civil strife, and other forms of political violence carried out by government and rebel forces, militias and paramilitary groups all involve armed conflict.[11] Before, during and after armed conflict, the proliferation of weapons and breakdowns in social controls, authority structures, and social support and other systems also contribute to violence within families and communities, as well as a range of deprivations that cause harm to civilian populations. Youth affected by armed conflict include those young people who are in the vicinity of, perpetrate, are victims of, and/or are otherwise directly affected by any of these forms of violence and their consequences and not just by open warfare.

Youth affected by armed conflict may be refugees, internally displaced persons (IDP) or returnees, or may never have fled their homes.[12] They may or may not themselves have been victims or perpetrators of physical violence. However, each has been affected in myriad ways by the instability and social, economic, political and psychological upheaval brought on or exacerbated by armed conflict, both during the hostilities and after the war has officially ended. Some of the effects of armed conflict on youth are visible, some are not; some are immediate, while others may only become apparent over time.

Not all young people in countries that have experienced armed conflict are necessarily "youth affected by armed conflict". In some cases, armed conflict is highly localized, leaving many of the country's inhabitants living outside these areas largely unaffected. Wars do have far-reaching social, economic and other effects outside of the areas in which their consequences are most directly felt, and many refugees and IDP flee conflict zones to areas otherwise untouched by war. However, a distinction is being made in the present context to zero in on youth who are most directly affected by armed conflict.

Demographics

Global data are not systematically collected on youth affected by armed conflict as a specific cohort, nor is there reliable information on their sex composition. Their numbers may be estimated, however, based on general population statistics and refugee and IDP statistics, which fluctuate.[13] If their share mirrors that of the average global youth population, young people between the ages of 15 and 24 comprise approximately 18 per cent of war-affected populations, and the number of females and males among them is almost equal.[14] However, because many countries affected by armed conflict and displacement have extremely youthful populations, the actual numbers of affected youth are likely higher than the global average would suggest.[15] In Pakistan, for example, which is still host to a million or more Afghan refugees, 60 per cent of the population is under the age of 25.[16]

The number of youth affected by armed conflict may not, by itself, provide a compelling rationale for focusing on youth and gender. After all, children under the age of 18 and adults aged 25 years and over each exceed youth in number globally. However, within war-affected societies, many of which are overwhelmingly young, youth are uniquely challenged to take on decision-making, caregiving and protective roles to ensure their own well-being and that of younger and older people. They are also looked to as defenders and maintainers of their culture, tasked with perpetuating traditional customs, values and practices. Further, the convergence of "large youth cohorts", high unemployment and other factors is believed to be associated with the onset of armed conflict, with the focus largely on young males in this context, raising important questions about the gender dynamics involved (Urdal, 2004).

THE ROLES OF YOUTH IN THE ONSET OF ARMED CONFLICT, SEEN THROUGH A GENDER LENS

Are youth prone to instigating and participating in armed conflict? What role does gender play?

Youth bulges

Much research on the involvement of youth in the onset of armed conflict focuses on the correlation between armed conflict and the existence of demographic "youth bulges", which occur when young people constitute an unusually large share of the overall population. This research is increasingly influencing how youth and conflict is framed as a global issue. It is argued that the mere existence of a youth bulge does not guarantee armed conflict, but that when other key factors are also present, the possibility of such conflict increases. Some of these additional factors include a high level of unemployment among youth, which fuels grievances among them; economic stagnation, which worsens periods of unemployment for youth; rapidly increased access to education, which can lead to stronger youth expectations for jobs and political and social influence that do not correspond to the actual opportunities available; and limited possibilities for migration, which means there is no safety valve through which countries might relieve unemployment-related pressures and defuse youth discontent. One study finds that the "combination of youth bulges and poor economic performance can be explosive" (Urdal, 2004).

Although all young people are presumably included in analysis of the significance of youth bulges, findings focus mainly on the lives and behaviour of male youth. One researcher categorically states the following: "Generally speaking, the people who go out and kill other people are males between the ages of 16 and 30" (Steinberger, 2001).[17] While males seemingly play a central role in comparison with females, a gender analysis of why male youth are the predominant actors in fomenting and carrying out armed conflict is strikingly absent from the youth bulge research. One important fact is that only limited numbers of males within the overall population of male youth participate in fighting forces. What explains the absence of most male and female youth from fighting forces despite their comprising the bulk of the youth bulge? Are they supportive of the onset of armed conflict in other ways? If not, what are they doing, and what happens to the voices of those who wish to be heard? These and many other important questions arise when a gender analysis is applied to research on youth cohorts and youth involvement in the onset of armed conflict.

If unemployment or the lack of access to resources generally affects females more than males, why are females not more apt than males to pick up weapons during economic downturns?[18] If, as some researchers believe, a higher level of educational attainment, when met with better job opportunities, tends to reduce the risk of armed conflict, why do large cohorts of uneducated female youth, who in general have had more limited access to educational opportunities, not pose a greater risk to stability than do males? Among highly educated young people, why do more males foment armed conflict? Why do the majority of males resist the temptation to engage in such conflict?

It should be noted that the onset of armed conflict also occurs during post-conflict periods. By the time a conflict is officially declared over, some young people may have achieved high levels of solidarity with one another and may have even greater access to weapons. Post-conflict societies are also usually economically devastated and face major challenges in rebuilding infrastructure. Do youth roles in the onset of armed conflict change in post-conflict situations? Is it easier or more difficult for males and females seeking to address their concerns to establish forums for effective, peaceful action in the post-conflict period?

These questions are raised to suggest a wider diversity of youth experiences in the onset of armed conflict than are accounted for in youth bulge analysis and to warn against the pitfalls of gender and youth stereotyping. The limitations associated with youth bulge analysis argue strongly for the adoption of holistic approaches to youth protection and development that take into account gender roles and dynamics, along with a host of other relevant factors. Youth bulge analysis does conclude, very plausibly, that when there are large numbers of young people placed under pressure to ensure their individual and/or collective survival and identity at a pivotal time in their lives involving the assumption of responsibility and status, they will seek diverse ways to cope, with some choosing armed conflict.

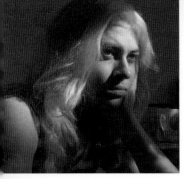

Gender and other dynamics associated with cycles of conflict are not fully considered in the youth bulge research. In failing to incorporate these dynamics, such research risks are stigmatizing all male youth as potential violent actors and female youth as passive victims; placing male experiences of deprivation and political and social marginalization at the centre of analysis and action surrounding youth and armed conflict and positing them as representative of female experiences; focusing on armed soldiering as the chief concern of youth affected by armed conflict, to the exclusion of the majority of other youth experiences; bypassing important opportunities to recognize and support constructive youth coping and activism; and finally, neglecting to address the root causes of conflict (including gender inequality) at the structural, cultural and other levels. Female and male involvement in violence, as well as in peaceful civil organizing and activism, is explored further in the next section.

YOUTH EXPERIENCES IN ARMED CONFLICT AND POST-CONFLICT SITUATIONS

What happens to male and female youth when armed conflict is under way and after it is officially over? What does this mean for these young people and their societies?

Moving beyond gender and youth stereotypes

Armed conflict rips apart the fabric of societies. People are killed, families are torn apart, communities are displaced and divided, infrastructure is destroyed, and support systems crumble. Under intense and often deliberate pressure from warring parties, social roles and norms undergo rapid change. In the process, youth are shown to be both vulnerable and capable because of their stage of development and the important gender and other roles they play in society. Youth are at once targets, perpetrators and survivors of violence and other rights violations in the upheaval of war.

Overall, youth are more likely than young children to be forcibly recruited into fighting forces; to suffer sexual violence; to miss out on educational opportunities; to head households and/or be forced to generate a livelihood for themselves and others with little support or training; to become pregnant (if female) and have little access to reproductive health-care information or services; to become teen parents; and to contract sexually transmitted infections (STIs), including HIV/AIDS, without access to prevention information or support for recovery (Lowicki, 2000). These experiences occur in a variety of settings, including refugee and IDP camps, urban areas, and rural villages and towns—and within fighting forces.

Apart from becoming pregnant and having specific reproductive health needs, both female and male youth may endure any or all of the experiences listed above to varying degrees depending on gender norms and the specific context of the conflict. The nature and dynamics of their experiences are similar in many ways but very different in others. For example, though males and females participate in fighting forces as combatants, females are more likely than males to also be used as sex slaves by commanders. By contrast, males may be forced to commit acts of sexual violence against females or males. Both sexes miss out on education in huge numbers. However, as described below, females are worse off, on average, and the consequences for them are often different. Females may be forced into early marriage and/or sexually exploited as a result of lost education. Males may also be forced into exploitative labour, but are less likely than females to be forced into sexual labour.

In these and many other ways, armed conflict often feeds on and worsens pre-existing gender divides. Amid the breakdown of social supports and controls, and with the advent of lawlessness, gender inequalities are often exploited, and impunity for gender-based violence is likely to prevail. Many males take advantage of the gender roles and secondary status of females and intensify discriminatory and abusive practices. From the increased sexual violence against them to the even deeper denial of access to resources and opportunities, females are often more brutally oppressed and abused during wartime, especially when they are refugees or IDP. At the same time, expectations of males as fighters and aggressors (and in other capacities) are also exploited. As conflict and power struggles among males progress, many are killed or find their options, resources and freedoms diminished or taken away. This fuels domestic abuse against females as males attempt to reassert their power, authority and perceived rights in other areas of their lives.

As indicated above, the violence associated with armed conflict is not confined to the battlefield. It also occurs within homes and communities, in part as a result of social upheaval and widening gender divides. Many abuses against children, young people and adults also occur, and even increase (especially for females), after conflicts have been officially declared over. The post-conflict period is often characterized by widespread lawlessness, corruption, attempts to seize power and control, and continued social upheaval. It is a time when old and new norms that subjugate females and stratify hierarchies among males may be reinforced. As roles, structures and systems are redefined, injustice may prevail, with marked increases in domestic and other violence against females and the harassment and intimidation of males.

At the same time, as bad as it is, armed conflict sometimes provides females and males with new opportunities to reshape their lives and relationships amid rapid social change. Gender roles are challenged and transformed by conflict, and some gender divides may be mitigated. For example, girls who were previously unable to go to school may be given the opportunity to do so in refugee camps. Females may become key family and community decision makers in the absence of males. Some males may have become activists for gender equality. These new opportunities may sometimes lead to additional gender divides, however, both during and after conflict, as females and males assume new roles and engage in new practices, only to encounter enormous resistance. For example, many Afghan refugees fled Taliban rule in order to secure education for girls. They and others have worked to expand this progress in post-conflict Afghanistan but often face setbacks. Recently, the Godah girls' school was set on fire in an attempt to intimidate students and organizers.[19]

Similarly, age divides may grow during armed conflict and in the post-conflict period as adults fail young people and the latter must act to fill gaps in support. Youth often lose respect for adults and adult-run institutions and systems that betray and abuse them instead of protecting and supporting them. Young people are forced to take on enormous responsibilities, caring for themselves and others with little support to ensure their survival

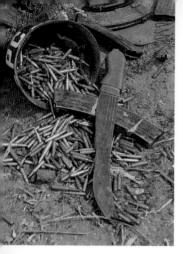

and recovery. Some develop strong leadership skills within fighting forces and attain high levels of authority that they are not always prepared to relinquish upon the cessation of fighting. Others, forced to provide for themselves in other ways, cannot afford to be side-lined in community action aimed at recovery, as their livelihoods are often at stake. Tension frequently exists between adults and youth as a result of role reversals, and as youth are stigmatized as uneducated, disrespectful or potentially violent. Young people continue to be marginalized from decision-making processes that affect their lives.

New opportunities emerge to support the rights and roles of young people as they actively cope with their circumstances in conflict and post-conflict situations. Some of their coping strategies are ultimately destructive to themselves and others, but with the right support can be transformed into critical life skills essential to individual and community recovery. Most, however, seek constructive ways of coping. Youth affected by armed conflict increasingly rely on peer support, and some form organizations, groups and associations that address a range of youth and community concerns. Some do so with help from supportive adults, bridging the gap between generations. Females participate in this organizing but are usually disadvantaged in terms of the range of leadership roles they may assume. In this context and many others, young people perpetuate gender and age-based inequalities. However, both male and female youth play important roles as mentors and activists, helping to improve the lives of younger children, members of their own age group, and others. Good practice acknowledging the value of supporting youth capacities, participation and leadership in and after armed conflict is also emerging.

The subsection below explores some of the ways in which youth and gender norms undergo dynamic change in armed conflict, revealing patterns and diversity that challenge purely stereotypical interpretations of gender, youth and armed conflict. Young people's experiences of violence, including murder and wounding, youth participation in fighting forces, and sexual violence, are described from a gender perspective. The impact of family upheaval on youth, the limited support for their education and health, and youth coping strategies are also viewed through a gender lens. Youth emerge as central agents in their own protection and care and as pivotal social actors, essential to social cohesion, conflict prevention and community recovery, who must be actively supported in ways that focus on their specific gender roles.

Young people's experiences of violence

All of the youth experiences of violence illustrated below involve gender differentials and reflect various forms of gender-based violence. Many forms of gender-based violence that young people suffer are brought on or exacerbated by armed conflict. While women and girls are not the only victims, they are the ones principally affected across all cultures because of their subordinate status in most societies (Ward, 2002).[20] Males are also strongly affected by gender-based violence, both as victims and as perpetrators, in ways that are often overlooked.

Gender-based violence is not experienced exclusively by male or female children, youth or adults. It exists along a continuum of violence and affects both sexes and all age groups, varying according to the circumstances. Although comprehensive statistics do not exist, it is believed that the number of women over the age of 24 who experience gender-based violence as a result of war is higher than the corresponding numbers of younger females (aged 15-24 years), males, or young children. Numbers, however, are not the principal concern, as the lives and experiences of all individuals in such situations are intertwined. The focus on youth as a cohort reveals important similarities and differences along age and gender lines that require distinct attention.

Murder and wounding

Both male and female youth are targeted by fighting forces for wounding and murder, but because of gender norms, males are often particularly affected. For example, in Kosovo in 1999, Yugoslav forces randomly abducted and killed ethnic Albanian adolescent boys and young and older men, fearing they might take up arms with the rebel Kosovo Liberation Army (KLA). Similarly, the KLA targeted ethnic Serbian and Roma males. Each group sought to undermine the cohesion and survival of the other's ethnic society (Organization for Security and Co-operation in Europe, 1999). In a number of conflicts, fathers have been targeted for murder or disappearance, leaving male youth behind to care for themselves and their families. These young men are at times denied access to schooling and are harassed and beaten by police, who suspect them of being part of opposition groups (Amnesty International, 2000).

Adolescent boys and young men are principal targets for murder and wounding because they are central to the functioning of patriarchal communities. Power and wealth are negotiated and passed on to the next generation through them. Eliminating or incapacitating them interrupts these processes and leaves male-dominated groups and societies vulnerable to collapse. Males may also be targeted based on the belief that wars are traditionally fought between males.

Girls and young women are targets for murder and wounding as well, not only in connection with sexual and other violence, but also for political and other reasons. Females have been targeted for murder and disappearance by fighting forces for stepping out of traditional gender roles, challenging the authority of armed groups, and taking action in support of human rights (Amnesty International, 2004a).

Women and children also make up a significant proportion of civilian deaths occurring as a result of the deprivation caused or exacerbated by armed conflict. The perpetration of violence against female youth affects their entire societies in the ways described below and symbolizes the failure of males to protect their families and communities. Rationales for murder and wounding in conflict situations are not solely gender-based but involve many other factors such as ethnicity, political affiliation, displacement circumstances, and socio-economic status.

Youth participation in fighting forces

Despite the intense international focus on young people as armed actors, those who actually engage in armed violence in or after armed conflict comprise a relatively small share of the overall youth population.[21] Statistics have not been compiled on the numbers of young people aged 15-24 years who are members of fighting forces. However, it is known that members of this age group make up a significant proportion of such forces. Most studies on young people's involvement in fighting forces concentrate on children under the age of 18 in an effort to address the contravention of prohibitions against their use as soldiers.[22] Although some are very young, most of the world's estimated 300,000 child soldiers (both males and females) are actually adolescents and youth. Some of the young people in fighting forces, who are over the age of 18 and considered legal participants, entered as children and were unable to leave.

Although international attention is often focused on male participation in fighting forces, females are widely involved as well. Recent research on girl soldiers shows that between 1990 and 2003, girls under the age of 18 were part of fighting forces in 55 countries. In 38 of these countries they were involved in armed conflicts, most of which were internal wars (fought among forces within national borders). Girls from a number of these 38 countries also participated in international armed conflicts (fighting between countries) (McKay and Mazurana, 2004). The research indicates that the motivations, causes and specifics of their experiences are widely diverse, and explores how they are similar to and different from the experiences of males. Extreme misogyny in armed conflict often makes female experiences in fighting forces more difficult than those of males (McKay and Mazurana, 2004).

Many male and female youth join fighting groups because they believe in a cause and/or because they feel they have no other options to sustain themselves, as education and job opportunities decline in times of conflict. Many young people indicate that the lack of access to formal or informal education is one of the primary reasons they join armed groups (United Nations, 2004a). In fighting groups, they may be given food, protection, an identity and recognized responsibilities. Many others are forced to join these groups; they may be abducted or drafted and subsequently indoctrinated. Youth may be viewed as easy targets, as they are not fully mature and are easily manipulated by their captors. Males are often recruited because they are believed to be strong and/or because fighting is seen as a male endeavour. Youth involvement in war is supported and strengthened by the widespread availability of small arms and light weapons to both State and non-State actors (see box 8.2), and by the abuse of drugs to enhance risk-taking and control.

While males are stereotypically assumed to be stronger and better fighters than females, members of both sexes perform many of the same duties within fighting forces. Like males, females take on roles as combatants, spies, messengers, lookouts, medics and supply carriers. Often, however, females are also recruited to play other roles compatible with traditional gender expectations, serving as captive "wives" or sex slaves, mothers, cooks and domestic servants. They are not simply camp followers but instead perform a range of critical functions in sustaining the activities of the fighting group. Forced or not, both males and females contribute to the violence of armed groups, including the acts of gender-based violence that are committed against young people and others. These individuals face, and will eventually be placed in the position of having to overcome, the enormous stigma attached to their involvement in violence and their association with fighting forces, as their activities in this context are seen to be responsible for the destruction of cultural and societal norms.

Box 8.2

THE IMPACT OF SMALL ARMS AVAILABILITY ON YOUNG PEOPLE

The proliferation of small arms has a devastating impact on the lives of youth, contributing greatly to their involvement in conflict, to social upheaval, and to acts of gender-based violence and discrimination. Their destructive potential is reflected in the following:[a]

- In the majority of conflicts, small arms are the main instruments of war causing death, injury and destruction.

- Young people are recruited to join armed forces and suffer severe physiological trauma from being forced to kill and maim using small arms.

- Because small arms cause casualties on all sides of a conflict, their proliferation weakens traditional family and support structures for young people.

- Small arms proliferation leads to population displacement, taking young people away from their homes and communities.

- Small arms endanger public life and safety and can therefore interfere with the provision of basic necessities such as food, education and health care.

- Small arms can seriously undermine the delivery of humanitarian assistance.

- Small arms contribute to "a culture of violence in the affected area, where [they] are used to cultivate influence, reinforce authority, and symbolize value".[b]

- Small arms are used for violent and criminal activities during and after conflicts, contributing to added or continuing insecurity.

- Small arms are portable and simple to use and are therefore relatively easy for young people to carry and operate.[c] In various conflicts they have been used to force children and youth to commit acts that effectively sever their ties with their families and communities and leave them no option but to join the armed forces.[d]

[a] Rachel J. Stohl, "Under the gun: children and small arms", *African Security Review*, vol. 11, No. 3 (Pretoria: Institute for Security Studies, 2002) (available from http://www.iss.co.za/Pubs/ASR/11No3/Stohl.html).

[b] Ibid.

[c] Women's Commission for Refugee Women and Children, "Problems and solutions identified by adolescent researchers in northern Uganda" (Gulu Research Team report, 2001), in *Against All Odds: Surviving the War on Adolescents*, Participatory Research Study with Adolescents in Northern Uganda (May-July 2001), p. 23.

[d] Stohl, loc. cit.

Challenges for male and female soldiers in post-conflict reintegration are similar in some ways and very different in others. Former child and youth soldiers need assistance reconnecting with their families and communities, medical care, a new and accepted identity (including as students in school or vocational training), and a means to sustain themselves. They are often extremely frustrated and at risk of experiencing ongoing protection problems when they do not find opportunities to fulfil their potential and use the skills and strengths they developed while members of fighting forces, and when they no longer command authority or resources.

As described later in the chapter, girls and women in fighting forces are often left out of disarmament, demobilization and reintegration (DDR) programmes, with important consequences for their protection and well-being. Overlooked and without support, they may be forced to remain with their captors, ostracized from their societies, or pushed into early marriage or prostitution, at times to support children born in captivity. They are also often left without psychosocial and medical care critical to their recovery. Demobilizing male youth are at risk of psychosocial distress, community stigmatization, re-recruitment and involvement in illicit activities if their needs are inadequately met.

Sexual violence

Sexual violence encompasses acts ranging from unwanted touching to wounding and mutilation, rape, sexual slavery, forced pregnancy, forced prostitution, and trafficking for sexual purposes. Rape victims may also be beaten and/or murdered. Rape is frequently used as a weapon of war by fighting forces not only to torture the individuals targeted but also to terrorize and destabilize their communities. Revelations of abuse can lead to stigmatization, blame of the victim, further physical harm, family rejection, the destruction of marriage prospects, health problems, and other serious consequences. Fearing such repercussions, survivors often remain silent and continue to suffer without the support they need for their psychosocial and physical recovery. Gender-based violence prevention and response systems are also often weak owing to social, cultural, legal and other constraints, and to the upheaval caused by war.

Stereotypically, females are perceived as victims and males as perpetrators of sexual violence. Although this is the general pattern, there are important exceptions.

Female youth and sexual violence

Generally speaking, though very young children and even babies may be affected, adolescent girls and young women are more likely than younger children and males to be sexually abused and exploited in armed conflict and post-conflict situations as gender roles are polarized. Such violence is frequently an intensification or continuation of violence experienced by girls and women and tolerated by their societies in peacetime. As they physically mature, girls and young women are often viewed as sexual objects and represent the wealth, cultural identity and future of their families and communities. Sexual violence against females may be random and capricious. It may also be systematic. Taking a woman's virginity or honour (and thus her value for marriage) and forcibly impregnating females are forms of "ethnic cleansing" affecting multiple generations. They undermine social identity and bonds, as well as family and community wealth and cohesion.

A number of recent examples provide a better understanding of the situation on the ground. During the conflict in Rwanda, the mass rape and sexual mutilation of Tutsi women and girls, and the deliberate transmission of HIV to them, were encouraged by Hutu extremists. In Bosnia and Herzegovina, women and girls were publicly raped prior to the expulsion of Muslim populations, and some were forcibly impregnated (Ward, 2002). The United Nations Office for the Coordination of Humanitarian Affairs estimated that between October 2002 and February 2003, approximately 5,000 women and girls were raped by fighting forces in South Kivu in the Democratic Republic of the Congo. Some were also deliberately injured in other ways, or even killed. It is believed that thousands of women and girls have been abducted or forced by desperate poverty to become sex slaves or front-line fighters. The victims in situations such as those described above, many of whom fear they have contracted HIV, have little or no support for their physical and psychosocial recovery and lack access to the mechanisms through which they might seek justice (Amnesty International, 2004b).

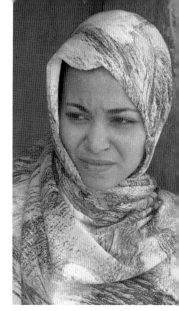

Refugee and internally displaced women and children, especially heads of household and young people who have lost or been separated from their families, are at particular risk of sexual violence. This violence occurs during their flight from or return to their homes, and in refugee camps and urban settings. Perpetrators may be bandits, members of government or other fighting forces, border guards, humanitarian aid workers, security personnel, members of host communities, or fellow refugees or IDP, including youth, teachers, neighbours or religious leaders.

Because refugee women and children often have limited means to sustain themselves and lack legal and physical protection, they are less able to assert their rights and therefore face a greater risk of sexual abuse and exploitation. Many resort to trading sex for food, protection or other services. Adolescent girls and young women are often placed in jeopardy by camp life and the roles they play in such settings. For example, they may suffer sexual violence as they collect wood or water to prepare food or as they carry out household chores or care for others (World Health Organization, 2000; United Nations High Commissioner for Refugees, 1999).

While all females may face gender-based violence in armed conflict and post-conflict situations, the specific threats and consequences are differentiated by age and by social and other circumstances. Older women may already be married and risk losing their families, shelter and community standing should the sexual violence they have suffered be revealed. They may even be labelled adulterers and murdered. Young female victims of sexual violence run the risk of never marrying, losing schooling opportunities, or being forced to marry their assailants. They may have fewer means than older women to help themselves. Younger females are more likely to contract STIs and experience maternal mortality. All survivors of sexual violence face lifelong psychosocial damage, and some may commit suicide.

Government, customary and other authority structures may no longer be functioning and therefore be unresponsive to, or even complicit in, sexual abuse and exploitation. In northern Uganda, child and youth "night commuters" walk miles every evening to town centres to sleep, fearing rebel attacks in their inadequately protected villages and IDP camps. Along the way and in sleeping spaces, females are especially at risk of sexual violence (Lowicki and Emry, 2004). In Afghanistan, under the rule of the mujahideen, rape and sexual harassment of women in Kabul were commonplace (Ward, 2002).

At times, international humanitarian personnel sexually abuse and exploit members of the local population, compounding the misery of the women and girls they are meant to protect. Experiences in the Democratic Republic of the Congo show that when faced with deprivation, both females and males often cope by engaging in prostitution. In 2004, the United Nations Office of Internal Oversight Services (OIOS) investigated 72 allegations of sexual misconduct by United Nations military personnel and civilian staff stationed in the Democratic Republic of the Congo (68 and 4 cases respectively). An OIOS report released on 5 January 2005 noted that "sexual contact with peacekeepers occurred with regularity, usually in exchange for food or small sums of money" (United Nations, 2005). The allegations involved women both under and over the age of 18, and in the cases that could be substantiated, most of the victims identified were between the ages of 12 and 16. Most of the encounters were facilitated by Congolese children and youth 8 to 18 years of age, and a few by young men aged 20-25 years (United Nations, 2005; Fleshman, 2005).

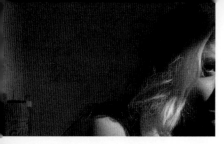

OIOS clearly identified youth, poverty, displacement and family loss or separation as key vulnerability factors for sexual abuse and exploitation or its facilitation. Investigators observed the following: "Most of the victims and witnesses are extremely vulnerable, not only because of their youth, but also because they are living alone, with other children or with older relatives in extended families who are unable to provide for them. The victims and a significant number of the boys are not in school because they cannot afford the fees" (United Nations, 2005, para. 31). The OIOS report also named job scarcity, an inadequate food supply, and a paucity of programmes to assist women and children as other key environmental factors in the abuse of young people. In this example, male and female youth facing similar circumstances found ways to cope within the limitations imposed by gender norms. Gaps in the monitoring and enforcement of restrictions on abuses by peace-keepers and others are further examined in a later section of this chapter.

Female genital mutilation

Many young females are exposed to a harmful traditional practice known as female genital mutilation (FGM), a social convention that involves the ritual cutting of female genitalia. The physical and psychosocial effects of FGM vary greatly depending on the nature and extent of the procedure and the cultural context (Yount and Balk, forth-coming).[23] Comprehensive information on how armed conflict affects FGM is not available. However, the upheaval caused by armed conflict certainly has an impact, given that FGM is a socially determined practice. Evidence from at least two regions suggests different scenarios: in the case of Sierra Leone, war may have led to a temporary decline in the practice; in Kenya, it may have contributed to an increase. In both places, new opportunities to end FGM or improve its safety emerged through education and community action.

During the hostilities, many girls and young women in Sierra Leone did not undergo FGM as part of the ceremonies associated with entry into women's Secret Societies because of massive displacement and devastated livelihoods.[24] In post-war Sierra Leone, there has been a resurgence in the practice, in part owing to the efforts of women who profit from it. Some young females have been abducted and held by Secret Society members until their families pay for the elaborate ceremonies. The issue is very politicized, and few within the Government or other authority structures will intervene. In other cases, young women and their families seek out the ritual to ensure their full participation in the social life of the community and as a way to gain reacceptance into society and establish the young woman's marriageability following a return from fighting forces. At the same time, many females are now interested in ending the practice or making it safer, having received information on its risks from reproductive health and gender-based violence programmes (Lowicki-Zucca, 2004a; Lowicki and Pillsbury, 2002; Yount and Balk, forthcoming).[25]

In the Dadaab refugee camps in Kenya, efforts to end FGM among Somali refugees backfired. When the first case against FGM was prosecuted in the camps in August 2002 under Kenyan law, refugee and local community members held demonstrations to protest what they saw as suppression of their cultural and religious rights. Not long after, Somali Bantus took further action to skirt the law when those in line for resettlement to third countries performed the procedure on girls as young as one and two in order to avoid further legal prohibitions. Refugee families that have banded together to ensure their girls do not undergo FGM have faced major reprisals. Some girls are barred from attending school, harassed, and risk never marrying (Munala, 2003).[26]

The United Nations and many Governments and non-governmental organizations (NGOs) have consistently and repeatedly condemned the practice of FGM. The issue is explicitly addressed in the United Nations Declaration on the Elimination of All Forms of Violence against Women, adopted in 1993.[27] Successfully challenging the practice of FGM requires a holistic approach that includes implementing and enforcing legislation, raising awareness about the harmful effects of FGM, and involving the various stakeholders at levels ranging from the community to the State (Amnesty International, 1998).

Male youth and sexual violence

Males may also be victims of rape and other forms of sexual abuse, and social taboos governing their ability to seek help are often more restrictive than those facing females. As is the case with females, sexual violence against males has the power not only to devastate the victim but also to destabilize society as a whole, given the prevailing gender norms. Perpetrators exert personal power over their male victims, often abusing positions of authority. When perpetrated by an opposition group, the abuse and humiliation inflicted serves to undermine the power and authority of all males in the family, community or society targeted. Although sexual abuse principally represents an expression of power and control rather than an effort to achieve sexual gratification per se, stigmas against homosexuality and the loss of power to another male are so strong that males may be much less inclined than females to come forward and seek justice, reparations, or help with recovery. The few services that exist for survivors of gender-based violence rarely address the needs of males (World Health Organization, 2000).

Rape and other forms of sexual coercion to which males may be subjected take place in the home, within the workplace, at school, on the street, in the military, during war, and in prisons and police custody. However, little reliable information is available on the extent of sexual violence against males. Although it is known to be less prevalent than that perpetrated against females, it remains largely unacknowledged and is believed to be vastly underrepresented. Some evidence suggests that males are particularly vulnerable in certain settings and contexts, including all-male institutions such as prisons or schools, and in armed conflict (World Health Organization, 2002). In settings in which male access to females is highly controlled or absent, risks of sexual violence increase for males (Lowicki, 2002). Often, males are forced by fighting groups to commit criminal acts against which there are extreme social taboos, including raping their mothers or sisters (Lowicki and Pillsbury, 2002).

Little has been done to identify or address the sexual abuse of males in conflict and post-conflict situations, and little action has been taken to further understand and better address the root causes of the perpetration of gender-based violence by males. In northern Uganda, when male youth began increasingly to harass and rape female night commuters in their communities, no one asked them why they were doing it. Subsequent interviews with some of the young men revealed a series of specific breakdowns in social support for and supervision of males that had led to the abuses. While some appeared simply opportunistic, other males revealed frustration with elders who no longer provided guidance and with the breakdown of traditional systems for meeting females and finding a bride. The males indicated that in the absence of opportunities to participate in traditional rites of passage, they had sought out alternative means of marking their transition to manhood, with little thought of the consequences for females (Lowicki and Emry, 2004). Additional attention to the social dynamics surrounding male sexuality and the roles of males as victims and perpetrators would reveal new avenues for prevention and care.

Impact on marriage patterns

Girls, in particular, are often subjected to early or forced marriages owing to the increased pressure armed conflict places on many families to make ends meet. When societies experience intense economic pressure, cultural practices become distorted. The time for marriage is often brought forward so that the bride's dowry may be acquired sooner rather than later, and some families effectively sell off their daughters for additional income. The vulnerability of girls is increased by their lack of economic, political and social independence. Girls and young women heading households are particularly at risk of early marriage, as they often have insufficient resources to care for themselves and any dependants, given the limited options available to them. Early marriage tends to be associated with dropping out of school, a range of health problems linked to early pregnancy and sexual activity, and ongoing dependence on males. Problems may also arise within the girl's new family when she is unable or unwilling to perform tasks as well as expected, having lost key years of preparation. This may lead to disputes and further physical abuse of the girl.[28]

Poverty and a lack of income may place males at a disadvantage within the family, seriously affecting their marriage prospects. For example, in some cultures, marriage requires the transfer of cattle to the family of the bride. Cattle represent the wealth and history of the family. Young refugee males may not be able to obtain cattle, and may therefore be unable to marry. Some are compelled to steal cattle, to make dangerous journeys in and out of conflict-affected areas to procure them, or to satisfy their desire for a wife through other, potentially forcible, means.[29]

Generating a livelihood

As family and other support systems break down in armed conflict, young people face major pressures to generate resources to ensure their own (and often others') survival and well-being. In the process, they face gender-specific protection problems and barriers to achieving self-sufficiency. When interviewed, young people in conflicts all over the world indicate that one of their main hopes is for self-sufficiency and to be able to provide for others. Insufficient livelihood is linked directly to exploitation and abuse, including sexual violence, early marriage, trafficking for sexual and other purposes, recruitment into fighting forces, and the spread of HIV/AIDS. Youth-headed households, which are most often run by females, are particularly at risk.

Armed conflict breaks down the structures and systems that normally prepare youth for economic roles and provide them with livelihood opportunities such as farming family lands or engaging in trade. Without these opportunities, many youth remain idle for extended periods and risk becoming involved in the types of destructive activities

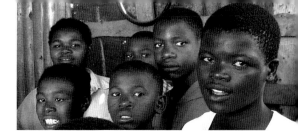

described above. Young people may also be forced into non-traditional roles. In many post-war societies, females have no choice but to take on traditional male livelihood roles, often becoming farmers or traders. Some youth may obtain a formal education while living as refugees, and upon returning home may no longer be interested in assuming traditional labour roles or observing established gender norms.

Youth who have managed to acquire a formal education or vocational skills are often challenged to find a market for their talents. In some cases, too many young people are provided with the same skills and cannot be accommodated in existing local labour markets. Markets are often weak in post-conflict environments, and poor infrastructure curtails trade and other opportunities. Youth may lack the tools, start-up capital, and basic business and entrepreneurship skills needed to set themselves up in a trade. Informal and semi-formal livelihood opportunities for young people are often neglected as possible starting points for economic development support. Further, advantage is rarely taken of new opportunities to break down gender barriers in employment, and it may be particularly difficult for females to gain full access to a range of employment options. The livelihood support programmes that are in place for women do not always address the particular capacity-building needs of adolescent girls and young women.

DDR programmes arguably represent the largest systematic attempts to address youth livelihood challenges in immediate post-conflict situations, but they answer only a small portion of the need and are often incomplete. Females, in particular, are often neglected. In development planning, too little attention is given to gender divides in employment, and inadequate account is taken of youth employment needs as they relate to education. Without economic support or opportunities, youth are placed in the position of being unable to provide for themselves or the next generation. These circumstances are particularly debilitating for females, many of whom are responsible for the care of younger children and others, as they become even more vulnerable to abuse and exploitation. Gaps in economic and social development support for young people also contribute to urbanization, emigration, and the increased exploitation of youth and their labour. Further, as stated previously, the existence of large numbers of unemployed youth constitutes a risk factor for further armed conflict.

Obtaining an education

Youth view education as essential to peace and economic development and to their own protection and personal development. However, in spite of the critical roles they play in their communities in and after armed conflict, they are more likely than young children to miss out on education opportunities essential to their well-being. Opportunities for education may be scarce even under normal circumstances but frequently become even more elusive for youth a result of armed conflict. Many young people are forced to forgo formal education because they have taken on new livelihood and caregiving responsibilities or are considered too old to make up the missed education. For financial and other reasons, few young people are able to complete secondary school in situations of armed conflict, and education interventions do not always adequately target the specific education needs of youth. In the absence of formal education, youth have few opportunities to obtain vocational skills training or other education when they need it most (Sinclair, 2004).[30]

Girls and young women without adequate educational opportunities face serious threats to their safety and security. Those who are in school are often required to drop out if they are forced into early marriage, become pregnant, or are heading households. They do not receive health education that would improve their care of themselves and others. Without skills training, their opportunities for earning an adequate living are generally more limited than those for males. As heads of household, they are likely to initiate or perpetuate a cycle of economic poverty and poor health that will affect the next generation. Out-of-school girls and boys typically have fewer opportunities to learn life-saving information about HIV/AIDS, landmines and other issues that may be critical to their survival.

Education provided within the framework of DDR programmes is largely targeted at males and represents an essential security tool, as it offers an immediate alternative to participation in fighting forces and a means through which young people can secure community acceptance and establish new roles and identities. Although there are many successes, those programmes that are poorly resourced leave demobilizing youth disappointed, disillusioned, and with few additional opportunities.

Overall, in comparison with males, females are consistently at a greater disadvantage in obtaining access to education and are often bypassed in DDR programmes. Girls face multiple barriers to education. When resources are scarce and families must choose which of their children to send to school, boys are given priority over girls. Available data show that gender-based differentials must be understood in the larger context of widespread educational deprivation affecting all youth in and after armed conflict.

A global survey on education in emergencies reveals that among refugees, enrolment generally begins to decline for both males and females after the first grade (*see figure 8.2*). Average differences between male and female enrolment remain fairly steady as both groups become less and less represented. Although the gap between female and male enrolment widens in later grades, these figures represent a very small number of refugee youth overall. The survey results for Pakistan indicate that in 2002, only around 4 per cent of the 194,000 refugee children and adolescents enrolled in school were in secondary education; 30 per cent (or around 2,300) of these older students were female, and 70 per cent (5,400 students) were male. At the time of the survey, Pakistan was host to more than 1 million refugees, at least half of whom were children and youth (Bethke, 2004).[31]

The most reliable statistics available on education in emergencies are compiled for refugees. Education opportunities for IDP are known to be much worse. Clearly, access to education remains extremely poor for both males and females affected by armed conflict. In post-conflict settings, reconstruction efforts tend to be focused on the rehabilitation of formal primary education systems serving mainly younger children in the eligible age group. Young people require a range of educational opportunities including formal primary, secondary and tertiary schooling; accelerated learning or "catch-up" classes; vocational training; entrepreneurship and business skills development; instruction to achieve functional literacy; and various types of non-formal and informal education ranging from sports and recreation to peace, health, conflict transformation and leadership education. Life skills, or values for living, cannot be overlooked in any educational context.

While young people view education as central to their protection and well-being, learning environments are not always safe, and an education does not always guarantee better life prospects or a sustaining livelihood. Corporal punishment, sexual abuse, and exploitative labour conditions are only a few of the challenges that may be faced in a variety of formal and non-formal educational settings. As mentioned previously, youth in refugee situations are sometimes provided with a quality education that might otherwise have been unavailable to them. If they are given the opportunity to return home, young people also require guidance and opportunities to put their education to good use. Even with their new skills, many are unable to find employment in their home communities and must explore other alternatives, including migrating from rural to urban areas in search of wider opportunities. Girls also face barriers to putting their education to use during post-conflict reintegration, as they are often expected to return to their traditional gender roles and may not be considered for traditionally "male" jobs.

Figure 8.2
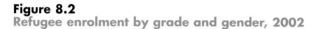
Refugee enrolment by grade and gender, 2002

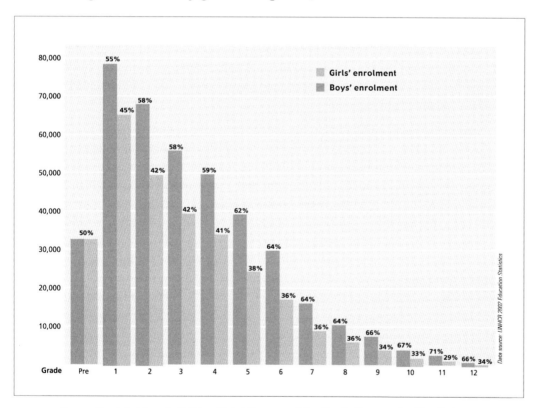

Source: Reprinted from L. Bethke, *Global Survey on Education in Emergencies* (New York: Women's Commission for Refugee Women and Children, 2004).

Reproductive health, including HIV/AIDS

The different forms of violence and deprivation youth experience in armed conflict have a dramatic effect on their health. The increased levels of poverty and violence and the lack of basic services in conflict settings exacerbate a wide range of youth reproductive health problems. Females are especially vulnerable because of their biological make-up and their exposure to targeted sexual violence and extreme deprivation.[32] Despite strong international commitments regarding the right to health care among women and girls, their reproductive health in and after armed conflict has been inadequately addressed. Even less attention has been given to the reproductive health of males, though they, too, face certain risks and can play an important role in improving the reproductive health of females.

The risks of sexual violence and exploitation, forced early marriage, and recruitment into fighting forces are especially high for the thousands of refugee youth who have lost or become separated from their parents or families as a result of war, HIV/AIDS or other causes.[33] Many young people also choose to have unprotected sex, increasing their risk of contracting STIs, including HIV. Females are particularly at risk of HIV infection owing to biological factors and the gender abuse and discrimination they face. Globally, the highest incidence of HIV infection among 15- to 24-year olds occurs in sub-Saharan Africa; three quarters of the young people in this age group who are living with HIV/AIDS in the region are female (Joint United Nations Programme on HIV/AIDS, 2004; Inter-Agency Standing Committee, 2004).

No direct causal relationship has been definitively established between a rise in armed conflict and increased HIV transmission. However, there are a number of recognized risk factors that apply to female youth in particular. Conflict exacerbates poverty, generally leading to an increase in sexual exploitation and young people's exposure to the virus. Women and girls are the least likely to command resources and must often rely on males for protection and services; with few options available, many exchange sex for food, shelter or other basic necessities. Girls and young women may even be sent by their parents to "receive gifts" from military personnel or others to support their families. Poverty also contributes to diminished access to both education (including information on HIV/AIDS prevention) and health care (including treatment for STIs), which increases the risk of HIV transmission. Social stigma and the lack of treatment options discourage youth from being tested, which would support further prevention. The increased use of drugs and alcohol by many young people in armed conflict impairs judgement and may contribute to sexual violence, also expanding the risk of HIV transmission to youth.[34]

The reproductive health problems faced by males include STIs, wounds affecting sexual and reproductive organs, and sexual dysfunction associated with sexual violence. The social stigma surrounding experiences of violence and sexuality in general often keep those who have been victimized from seeking assistance. Enhanced programme outreach efforts are needed to help boys and young men recover from sexual violence, to address any concerns they may have about reproductive health, and to strengthen their partnership role in ensuring that the reproductive health rights of girls and young women are respected.

Both male and female youth often have few sources of accurate information about sexual health owing to the breakdown of social, education and health systems and strong social taboos against discussing sex. Parents are often as ill informed as their children about reproductive health and sexuality issues, and most young people rely on the uninformed advice of peers when making decisions that affect their reproductive health. At the same time, they often lack the communication and negotiation skills to ensure safer sex with partners or to refuse sex. In some cultures, sex is not necessarily consensual, and females, especially, do not feel they have the right to refuse. In many cases, young people are unaware of and lack access to existing health services in emergencies and post-conflict situations, pointing to major gaps in youth outreach efforts among health providers.

Although young people have consistently expressed a strong interest in knowing their reproductive health rights and doing more to protect themselves, their participation in the design, monitoring and evaluation of reproductive health programmes remains limited. Further, little effort has been made by young people or reproductive health practitioners to determine the extent to which awareness-raising, life-skills and peer approaches induce behavioural change among youth and what factors are most important in different contexts. Many girls without education or economic alternatives say that even with information on reproductive health, they are still forced to marry early or to exchange sex for money, goods or services. Gender-based-violence programmes addressing the root causes of gender inequality and discrimination are not yet widespread, nor are youth-focused reproductive health programmes in emergency and post-conflict settings, though such initiatives are increasingly being developed and implemented.[35]

Youth coping and activism

In the face of myriad assaults on their well-being, youth affected by armed conflict actively cope with their circumstances. In taking on traditional "adult" roles and serving as soldiers, parents, heads of household, and labourers, young people push the boundaries of gender and youth norms and create new social roles for themselves that sometimes challenge existing gender and youth norms and inequalities. In many cases, however, they perpetuate established norms and inequalities, and opportunities to mitigate the latter are frequently lost. Too often, youth remain marginalized from family, community, national and international institutions and systems that do not recognize or support their critical contributions and roles.

Peer relationships become especially important to youth in areas affected by conflict. Young people turn to one another for comfort, companionship and support to fill gaps in their protection and care. They develop friendships and romantic attachments, and they organize formal and informal associations and groups. Internally displaced girls in Uganda find spaces to talk and relax by water pumps or when doing laundry or marketing. In refugee camps and towns in Albania, Kosovar refugee youth formed groups with Albanian youth and organized activities ranging from sports to protection monitoring (Bainvel, 1999). In Liberia, youth lead peer education campaigns, sharing health and other information. In Burundi, youth who have been orphaned or separated from family members band together to raise goats for income-generation and offer one another moral support. At times, international and local adult-run organizations facilitate youth activism. More often, though, youth come together on their own.

Some youth groups organize more formally and become focal points for youth activism, conveying their concerns to adults and other decision makers, as well as to their peers. Youth NGOs channel youth energy, voices and ideas into action to address a range of issues, including HIV/AIDS prevention and care, tolerance and peacebuilding, conflict prevention, gender sensitization, socio-economic development, good governance and more. In post-conflict Sierra Leone, for instance, hundreds of civil society youth organizations have been established. Many of them worked together with a receptive minister of youth to pass a national youth policy. Youth also form student and religious groups. Through these activities, youth build their capacities and assert new roles as key actors in humanitarian response and post-conflict reconstruction efforts.[36]

All of these peer activities help youth survive, secure psychosocial support, and feel more connected to their communities. Youth also care about the things they are achieving and have a vested interest in them. Their actions open doors to deeper discussion and collaboration with supportive adults. These new "peer ecologies", emerging out of the upheaval of conflict, are important starting points for working with youth and are indicative of the strengths and skills youth have developed to survive and recover from conflict.

In the process of taking on new and different roles, young people often transform gender and youth stereotypes, but they may also recreate them. Groups may be made up of all females, all males, or males and females together. Although females may attain some leadership positions, most mixed youth organizations are not headed by females. Because of their secondary status, females are not taken seriously in some patriarchal societies, and male leaders are seen as necessary to compete. However, females acting as advocates sometimes have greater access to decision makers than do males because they are viewed as less of a threat to male authority. Youth organizations may need to make stronger and more successful efforts to involve females, as recommended by international NGOs and other donors. In other cases, cultural norms may not permit females and males to interact. Females may lead all-female groups but not mixed groups.[37]

In spite of these and other gaps, girls and young women do at times play strong leadership roles, even if not as heads of organizations. In a number of settings, males and females have built strong working relationships, creating a new consciousness among themselves to work for gender equality. In one instance, the female co-founder of a youth organization has observed that just creating spaces for girls to sit together and talk about their concerns is an enormous achievement. The male co-founder agrees and says that one of the greatest challenges to addressing the concerns of all youth is addressing the root causes of gender inequality.[38] Over time, this group has been able to win the ear of government decision makers, but little follow-up action is taken.

Women's groups tend not to interact with youth groups or to actively support the roles of adolescent girls and young women within them. In part, this may be because women's groups take a narrower approach to gender activism and may not immediately see common ground with male-led youth NGOs. Women's groups often do not consciously address age-specific concerns of females or work to develop female youth leadership. Youth are sometimes able to find support through spiritual activities or from religious organizations administering educational, relief or other assistance programmes. Some of

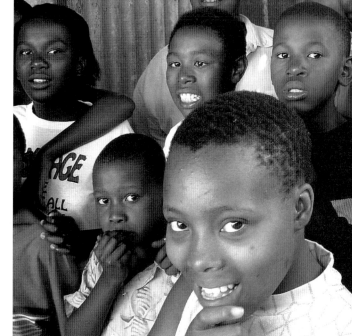

these organizations may help young people empower themselves through means such as girls' education and spiritual support. Often, however, such groups stratify structural and interpersonal gender divisions according to religious beliefs that legitimize male dominance.

In other instances, youth consolidate the power they have gained by establishing or participating in political parties. In Sierra Leone, some of the youth involved in the Revolutionary United Front (RUF) rebel group threatened to return to fighting if their concerns were not addressed. In post-war Kosovo, male leaders of various fighting groups formed political parties, simply transferring their power and influence to another arena in which they could exercise control. In these scenarios, male youth perpetuate existing political agendas. Some youth organizations are elitist and engage only the least marginalized young people, such as those in school.

Opportunities to bridge gender divides and reinforce the common ground between females and males are often lost, despite the strong consensus among youth about the key issues they are facing. In comparative research designed and conducted by youth in three countries affected by armed conflict, more than 2,000 young people were interviewed by their peers, and the findings indicated that males and females shared the same top concerns and offered many of the same solutions (Lowicki, 2004).[39]

The youth-led research revealed that complex sets of factors were working together to influence young people's overall protection and development, ranging from the prevalence of armed conflict and the availability of education, jobs and health care to love, gender equality, and respect and mentoring from parents, peers and others. The actions youth believed were necessary to support their protection and development varied greatly along gender, displacement, family status and other lines, according to the context. Beyond peace and the absence of armed conflict, youth named education, especially as it related to livelihood prospects, as key to their present and future well-being. Barriers to education and livelihood are often quite different for males and females and require different strategies to overcome. In efforts to address the root causes of problems facing youth and their communities, integrated approaches are needed that are informed and driven by both male and female youth so that a better understanding may be obtained of the unique challenges faced by each group (Lowicki, 2005; Newman, 2004).

Although there is growing international interest in youth as peacebuilders in the context of conflict prevention and recovery, most young people are not engaged in peacebuilding per se but are involved in activities that help to advance peace. They share an interest in political peace processes and targeted conflict transformation and resolution, but their attention and efforts are largely focused on ensuring their overall well-being and averting the root causes of war and human misery-including their own misery.

Despite young people's achievements and the key roles they play, youth rights and capacities are not adequately recognized in armed conflict or post-conflict situations. For instance, youth employment needs are not prioritized in development activities. Youth opinions are rarely sought, and young people are not integrated into leadership structures. More work is needed at the community and national levels to help youth find ways to bridge gender and age divides. Children, youth and adults of both sexes need spaces and processes that may be used to resolve tensions and achieve a better understanding of the realities of gender and youth dynamics, and why it may be impractical or impossible to revert to old norms. Adolescent girls and young women need targeted support to build their leadership capacities, including, when possible, in partnership with women's organizations and males. Many children, youth and adults are already working together to identify and apply creative ways to address gender and youth divides. Good practice should be developed and expanded.

Box 8.3 provides an excellent example of how children and youth in Colombia worked together and with others to draw international attention to the situation of children in armed conflict and to promote peace. The Children's Movement for Peace has been credited with helping to ensure that peace talks between the Government and leaders of a 35-year-long guerrilla insurgency were restarted (United Nations Children's Fund, 2005).

Box 8.3

YOUNG PEOPLE VOTE FOR PEACE IN COLOMBIA

In 1996, more than 2.7 million children and youth in different provinces all over Colombia, comprising the recently formed Children's Movement for Peace, participated in a special election known as the Children's Mandate for Peace and Rights. Their ballot incorporated 12 basic rights taken from the Colombian Constitution and the Convention on the Rights of the Child. Through their votes, the children communicated their three highest priorities: the right to enjoy life and good health, the right to peace and protection in war, and the right to love and family. One year later, inspired by the success of this initiative, 10 million adults (twice the usual voter turnout) held a national referendum known as the Citizen's Mandate for Peace, Life and Liberty, the results of which helped determine the outcome of the next presidential election (the winner, Andres Pastrana, ran on a platform for peace).[a]

Over 100,000 children have become active participants in the Children's Movement for Peace in Colombia, supported by UNICEF, the Red Cross and other human rights groups. In both 1998 and 1999, the Children's Movement was nominated for the Nobel Peace Prize, drawing worldwide attention to the situation of young people in armed conflict. The members of the Movement, many of whom come from deprived areas in conflict, have been actively promoting peace throughout Colombia. They have lost friends and family in the violence and have witnessed kidnappings and random killings, and they are determined to build a better future for themselves and the young people to come. Some members have faced death threats because of their work for the Peace Movement.[b]

Unfortunately, the impact of the Movement has deteriorated in recent years, and reports from Colombia indicate that adolescents are becoming increasingly marginalized and disenfranchised.[c]

---

[a] United Nations Children's Fund, "Promoting a culture of peace", a photo essay (available from http://www.unicef.org/girlseducation/23929_14675.html; accessed on 18 July 2005).

[b] Cable News Network, "The world's children: soldiers of peace" (available from http://www.cnn.com/SPECIALS/1999/children/stories/child.soldiers/#teens; accessed on 18 July 2005).

[c] Watchlist on Children and Armed Conflict, *Colombia's War on Children* (New York: Women's Commission for Refugee Women and Children, February 2004), p. 10.

ADDRESSING MULTIPLE CONCERNS AND MOVING FORWARD

How are gender, youth and armed conflict issues currently approached at the policy and programme levels? What are some of the ways forward?

This section highlights some of the more noteworthy achievements and gaps in efforts to ensure youth rights and gender equality in armed conflict and post-conflict situations. The examples are not fully representative of the wealth and breadth of experience and work relating to these issues, but are sufficient to strengthen arguments for improving holistic youth and gender approaches while also expanding youth and "women and girls" approaches.

Women's and children's rights agendas shape gender and youth approaches

Young people affected by armed conflict theoretically enjoy the full range of protections guaranteed under international, national and regional law and related policies and guidelines, including protection from violence and gender discrimination. Efforts to address youth and gender issues have largely straddled two somewhat parallel streams of policy and practice, one devoted to child protection and development, and the other to the protection and advancement of women. Each of these approaches is urgently needed to ensure ongoing support and protection of the rights of children and women, and there is a certain degree of overlap between them. However, as noted above, they often fail to adequately address the diverse age and gender concerns that arise or intensify during and after armed conflict. Gender approaches have tended to focus primarily on females, with limited age differentiation. Youth-related initiatives have not fit squarely into child- or adult-related programming, as the needs of young children and older adults are given priority. When youth or gender issues are addressed within these contexts, a stereotypical approach is often taken; for example, priority attention might be directed towards males as soldiers.

"Youth" bridges legal and customary interpretations of childhood and adulthood. As the legal age of majority is 18 in most contexts, individuals between the ages of 15 and 24 may qualify for international legal protection as children or adults. Young people under 18 years of age are protected under the United Nations Convention on the Rights of the Child, which contains provisions supporting the rights of war-affected children, including refugees (United Nations, 1989). Youth above and below the age of 18 are covered by similar provisions in the Universal Declaration of Human Rights, the International Covenant on Civil and Political Rights, the International Covenant on Economic, Social and Cultural Rights, and other instruments. Because they are not explicitly mentioned, however, youth are often "invisible" in both the interpretation and enforcement of these standards.

Most international legal instruments dealing with gender either explicitly address or are interpreted as addressing the situation of women. The Convention on the Elimination of All Forms of Discrimination against Women includes specific provisions relating to the situation of women in war and as refugees and implicitly covers adolescent girls and young women. Non-discrimination is also invoked in other treaties providing for the protection of adults and children affected by conflict, including the Convention relating to the Status of Refugees. In the implementation and enforcement of these and other commitments, the

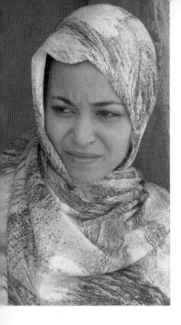

age- and gender-specific concerns and experiences of youth are not fully addressed together. Guidelines for the protection of refugee women and children provide limited information on the age-specific needs of youth and approaches for dealing with this group. In another example, while international commitments to achieving education for all have been made and include an emphasis on gender equality, efforts have largely been focused on achieving universal primary education, with little attention given to the educational needs of youth affected by armed conflict.

Efforts to identify and address specific youth and gender concerns are further complicated by the use of the terms "women and girls" and "women and children". In treaties and follow-up efforts relating to women's rights, reference is sometimes made to "women and girls", implying a continuum of female experiences. "Girls and young women" are often tacked on to discussions of women's rights, or assumed to be included, with little attention given to their distinct gender- and age-related experiences. Similarly, "women and children" are linked together in references to particularly vulnerable groups. There is a strong connotation here of children as women's dependants, invoking images of small children. Many certainly are, but the breadth of young people's experiences from early childhood through adolescence is not reflected in the terminology or, ultimately, in comprehensive action. Within the children's rights framework, references to "girls and boys" do not sufficiently differentiate adolescent/youth experiences. Programmes for children that serve only those under the age of 18 often create arbitrary distinctions between the experiences of youth under the age of 18 and those of young people over the age of 18.

Young people would benefit from more explicit declarations of their rights, and in efforts to advance the rights of women and youth, girls and young women would benefit from attention to their age- and gender-specific concerns.

Beijing and beyond

The Fourth World Conference on Women, held in Beijing in 1995, set the stage for concerted global action aimed at the achievement of women's rights. Young people involved in the Conference's vibrant youth programme produced the Youth Platform for Action. Among other things, the youth participants stated that the full impact of conflict situations on females of all ages should be acknowledged and researched.[40] Many elements of the Youth Platform have been pursued further. The Beijing Declaration and Platform for Action calls for initiatives in support of the rights of "women and girls", including those affected by armed conflict, and strong efforts have been made to increase support for girls' education in a variety of settings. However, follow-up has not intensively focused on or involved adolescents and youth.

Building on the Beijing Declaration and Platform for Action and the efforts of the United Nations General Assembly and others, the United Nations Security Council adopted resolution 1325 on women and peace and security in 2000. The resolution calls for the equal participation of women in all efforts to maintain peace and security and reaffirms the need to protect women and girls from human rights abuses, including gender-based violence. It also identifies a need to mainstream gender perspectives in conflict prevention, peace negotiations, peacekeeping operations, humanitarian assistance, post-conflict reconstruction and DDR initiatives (United Nations, 2000b).

Although women and girls are mentioned explicitly in Security Council resolution 1325, policy developments relating to gender, peace and security indicate that there have been only superficial attempts made to understand the specific implications of conflict for girls and young women and to involve them in peacebuilding. There has been a general failure to convey the meaning of Security Council resolution 1325 to girls and young women in conflict-affected countries and to work together not only with women's organizations but also with youth organizations on implementation and monitoring. Humanitarian action focused on women does not regularly incorporate differentiated approaches to adolescents and youth. In a recent study on gender, peace and security, the Canadian Peacebuilding Coordinating Committee calls for more careful use of the terms "women" and "girls" to ensure that the similarities and differences in their experiences are adequately conveyed. The Committee also recommends capacity-building efforts to ensure that girls and young women are able to participate more actively and effectively in peacebuilding and in policy and programme development and implementation (Kirk and Taylor, 2005).[41]

Women's groups, Governments and others working to implement Security Council resolution 1325 should take the necessary steps to ensure that the resolution has a visible impact on girls and young women affected by armed conflict (United Nations, 2000b). Gender, peace and security issues should be viewed from the perspectives of women and girls, as well as through a broader "gender lens", and what is learned through this process should guide policy decisions. Male and female youth (and not only older adult women) should have a place at the table in peace negotiations to address gender and other concerns. Increased coordination and commitment is also needed to ensure the implementation and enforcement of Security Council resolutions on children and armed conflict, with particular attention given to the complex gender dynamics characterizing the experiences of children and youth in and after armed conflict. Mentoring relationships between adult women and young women and girls should be strengthened, as should collaboration between women's groups and youth groups. Youth groups provide important opportunities for female empowerment as well as opportunities to engage males in action for gender equality. Existing youth groups represent a multiplicity of youth concerns and areas of interest and action, indicating that narrow conceptions of youth in conflict as victims or perpetrators of violence, or even as peacebuilders, are unfairly limiting.

Winnipeg and beyond

The actions described below, which have been undertaken both with and on behalf of children affected by armed conflict, have opened the door to increased action with and for youth. The momentum generated by the Convention on the Rights of the Child, Graça Machel's report on the impact of armed conflict on children, and the creation of the Office of the Special Representative of the Secretary-General for Children and Armed Conflict (OSRSGCAC) ushered in an era of increased global action focused on children affected by armed conflict. In 2000, the Government of Canada hosted the International Conference on War-Affected Children in Winnipeg. The Conference broke new ground by involving adolescents as central participants in the event and had a vibrant youth forum.[42] Young people from many different countries, including those affected by conflict, were also deeply involved in the United Nations Special Session on Children in 2002.

Governments, United Nations agencies, and others participating in the Winnipeg Conference made a number of commitments covering a comprehensive range of issues facing children affected by war. In the outcome document, adolescents are explicitly identified as a group requiring further attention and resources, and girls and women are singled out for targeted approaches. There is also a call for a sustained commitment to child participation in decision-making that affects their lives (Canada, no date). Although the meeting focused on the rights of children, youth participants were given the opportunity to prepare and present a youth statement in which they specifically identified themselves as "youth" and spoke of their concerns as children and young adults.

In principle, all the provisions of the outcome document of the United Nations Special Session on Children pertain to all children, including those affected by war; however, the needs of the latter group are more specifically addressed in a section on protection from armed conflict. Among other things, there is a call for the involvement of children in peace processes and for special attention to the vulnerabilities of girls (United Nations, 2002b). At both of the meetings just mentioned, the international community convened to address the needs of children, and while the young people present raised a number of critical youth issues, youth-focused initiatives were not explicitly recommended. In both cases, discussions and recommendations remained focused on "children", and gender was mainly interpreted as "girls".

The OSRSGCAC and other children's advocates working with the United Nations Security Council have been instrumental in ensuring the adoption of a series of important Security Council resolutions on children and armed conflict.[43] These unprecedented resolutions address a wide array of child protection and care issues ranging from ensuring humanitarian access to children in war zones to ending the forced recruitment of children into fighting forces. Girls constitute the major focus in references to gender concerns; various provisions address the needs of girls in DDR programmes and in actions to end gender-based violence and emphasize the need to ensure their access to humanitarian aid. The resolutions also call for young people's involvement in peacebuilding activities. Follow-up advocacy efforts have been strongest in the area of child soldiering. While this issue is extremely important, advocacy efforts must be broadened to address a range of other issues facing young people; in particular, action is needed to strengthen the capacity and reinforce the constructive roles of young people in humanitarian action. In efforts by the OSRSGCAC and others to develop effective monitoring, reporting and compliance mechanisms that will ensure the protection of children, attention should also be given to supporting youth roles and investigating the age- and gender-specific issues facing young people.

Field action supporting child participation in humanitarian programming has grown in the context of these achievements and has mainly involved adolescents and young adults. However, this work remains limited in terms of the extent to which it helps young people build their capacity as key actors informing and implementing a range of interventions affecting their lives over time. Youth organizations are still not regularly supported in ways that help them build the capacity they need to become key partners, using what they learn through engagement with their peers both inside and outside organized groups to inform, implement and evaluate humanitarian policies and actions that affect them. As a result, youth issues are still often poorly understood, and the potential of youth to become central actors in constructive social change, recovery and security is squandered.

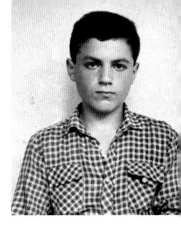

At times, support for youth leadership has been divisive, serving to pit young people against one another in pursuit of limited resources, as opposed to helping them improve cooperation. International agencies working in post-conflict Kosovo vied for access to existing youth organizations and created competition among them. As a result, collective youth voices were muffled in the early stages of reconstruction planning and action, with long-term effects on the actions taken to address their rights and roles through the transition to development. In other scenarios, the emphasis on youth as either peacebuilders or former or potential violent actors allows no room for recognition and support of the coping skills, strengths and interests youth have that constitute the key building blocks for their survival and societal recovery. Opportunities to build on transformations in gender norms among youth are also often lost.

Owing largely to the Organization-wide commitment to improving action for child protection, and more specifically to the efforts of dedicated staff at the various headquarters and country offices, United Nations agencies have made important strides in identifying and addressing adolescent and youth issues in their work. The UNICEF Adolescent Development and Participation Unit supports, from its headquarters in New York, various adolescent protection, education, health and other programmes. The Office of the United Nations High Commissioner for Refugees (UNHCR) has similarly demonstrated its commitment to addressing the particular needs and risks faced by youth and has, among other things, sponsored youth-led research and advocacy. Recently, the United Nations Development Programme (UNDP) conducted a review of its work with youth in conflict (United Nations Development Programme, 2005). However, there is no focal point for leadership on issues affecting youth in and after emergencies and no concerted effort to address the specific problems of young people in conflict situations as informed by a comprehensive framework for action.

Mainstreaming youth and gender

Arguments can be made both for mainstreaming youth and gender concerns and for engaging in targeted work with youth, women, girls, or other groups. Approaches that focus specifically on women, girls, or female youth are needed to ensure that the urgent gender issues affecting each of these groups are not diluted. However, the adoption of a broader gender approach makes it possible to address the full range of gender divides and to develop holistic approaches to prevention and response deriving from a better overall understanding of underlying causes. In either case, it is important to avoid simplistic approaches to female issues and to improve attention to male gender concerns and action with males on gender equality. Work to ensure that youth concerns are mainstreamed into broader national and international programmes can and should be matched with targeted action in support of age-specific programmes and policies that prioritize youth rights and capacities. Where possible and appropriate, youth and gender should be more closely linked in addressing issues of concern to young people, and these issues should be seen as extending across children's, women's and other agendas.

Mainstreaming processes involve transformations at many levels; it is not enough to simply incorporate girls, women or youth in existing activities. United Nations agencies and Member States have worked to develop gender mainstreaming plans and expand women's participation in humanitarian response. However, similar efforts have not been made to promote the involvement of children and youth affected by armed conflict (the stated approach of UNHCR represents one of the few notable exceptions). Policies and guidelines already in place would benefit from age-specific analysis, and from the establishment of implementation, monitoring and accountability mechanisms. Greater attention should also be given to prevention, enforcement and response.

Sufficient resources, a sustained commitment to coordinated action at the highest levels, and a broader understanding of youth and conflict issues are all required to ensure effective implementation, monitoring and follow-up. Assessments of gender mainstreaming in the Consolidated Appeals Process (CAP) reveal a need for improved gender analysis and sex-disaggregated data; however, age-disaggregated data are also needed to address the specific gender concerns of females and males at different stages of their lives (United Nations, 2004b). Support for programming targeted at women and children is consistently more forthcoming in CAP responses than that targeted at youth. Improved articulation of the rights of young people and promising practices indicating how best to work with them across women's, children's and other programmes would help change the situation.

Overall, little progress has been made in mainstreaming youth and gender perspectives in efforts to address the needs of war-affected populations. The Youth Employment Network (YEN),[44] an outcome of the Millennium Summit and Millennium Declaration, is an encouraging example of an attempt to mainstream youth in the area of employment at the international level. The YEN is receiving increasing support from national Governments; however, there has not yet been any real attempt to focus on youth employment and gender issues within conflict and post-conflict environments.

Youth and gender mainstreaming is particularly important in efforts to address sexual and other gender-based violence in conflict and post-conflict situations, given the relative vulnerability of both female and male youth. Some progress has been made in dealing with the sexual abuse and exploitation involving United Nations and other humanitarian assistance personnel, but major gaps remain. Many organizations have taken action to adopt the Core Principles of a Code of Conduct for Protection from Sexual Abuse and Exploitation, developed for humanitarian agencies by the Inter-Agency Standing Committee (IASC) Task Force on Protection from Sexual Exploitation and Abuse in Humanitarian Crises.[45] However, enforcement of the Code of Conduct remains difficult.

The OIOS, in its report on sexual abuse and other misconduct in the Democratic Republic of the Congo, noted that the "zero tolerance" policy of the United Nations had been undermined by "zero compliance", as the United Nations Mission in the Democratic Republic of the Congo (MONUC) had failed to put enforcement mechanisms in place (United Nations, 2005; Fleshman, 2005). New restrictions were imposed on MONUC and other peacekeeping staff, monitoring and evaluation efforts were strengthened, and in coordination with those countries contributing peacekeeping troops, changes were made in training, command and disciplinary approaches. Although Member States have expressed some concerns regarding disciplinary measures, they have not given the United Nations the authority to enforce rules or punish perpetrators; this remains the responsibility of the individual contributing countries (Fleshman, 2005).

Steps must be taken to improve coordination between women's and youth groups, international NGOs, the United Nations, and national Governments to curb sexual abuse and exploitation and to promote gender and age mainstreaming in other areas. Reference points must be created to more clearly define areas of priority and facilitate concerted action; in particular, there is a need for a comprehensive youth and armed conflict framework that reflects gender considerations, and an institutional focal point must be identified for coordinated action within the United Nations system. This focal point would work closely with NGOs and United Nations staff, as well as with women and youth, to more effectively assist those young people who are actively coping with a multitude of challenges on a daily basis with minimal support. The United Nations Office for the Coordination of Humanitarian Affairs is currently putting together a gender mainstreaming handbook that not only identifies specific actions that may be taken in different sectors, but also provides sets of impact indicators. These guidelines may be used to address some youth concerns.

Humanitarian and post-conflict reconstruction initiatives

Without strengthened support along the various tracks mentioned thus far, young people's concerns will not be adequately addressed in humanitarian response and policy and prevention efforts. Support for youth protection and development before, during and after armed conflict is not regularized and does not sufficiently address gender divides. When interventions are undertaken, they are not integrated in ways that engage all sectors effectively, and they often fuel competition between youth rather than building constructive solidarity among them. Some good practice addressing youth and gender equality issues in conflict situations is emerging and should be expanded (Lowicki, 2000; 2004). No comprehensive framework for action exists, nor is there a strong international consensus in this regard, making it difficult to address the multiple challenges youth face in diverse conflict and post-conflict environments.[46] Divisions between humanitarian and development agendas present further challenges.

The subsections below provide some additional examples of achievements and gaps, as well as various recommendations, relating to youth- and gender-focused humanitarian response, building on the previous examples relating to reproductive health, education, livelihoods and youth activism.

Lessons from gender-blind disarmament, demobilization and reintegration efforts

Significant strides have been made in improving DDR efforts with children and adults and along gender lines. However, promising practices are not adequately expanded and implemented in other regions. DDR in Sierra Leone is often touted as good practice; however, lessons from the experience, including the need for increased efforts to overcome major gender gaps, are still not fully applied. The Lomé Peace Accord, which ushered in opportunities for peace in Sierra Leone, specifically addressed child and gender concerns. UNICEF and child protection agencies made valiant efforts and ultimately reintegrated thousands of children and adolescents formerly with fighting forces. However, DDR in Sierra Leone was largely gender blind, and many demobilizing female children and youth did not receive the support they needed.

In Sierra Leone, a distinction was made in DDR efforts between "ex-combatants" and those recruited to serve a range of other purposes, making it particularly hard for females to gain access to formal reintegration support. An initial "cash for weapons" approach also placed females at a disadvantage, as males in fighting forces pulled weapons from females and others to consolidate access to forthcoming support during disarmament. Commanders were asked to attest to who had participated in the forces, barring many more females from inclusion. UNICEF made additional assistance available to girls, as it included "camp followers" among the child programme beneficiaries. This and other support came late, however, and with few alternatives, many girls ended up in sex work or remained with their captors. In an effort to address such gaps, NGOs, United Nations agencies and others are developing new expertise on the specific gender needs of demobilizing young people; some, for example, are working with females with children born in captivity and their families to address their special needs (Lowicki and Pillsbury, 2002).[47]

In connection with these and other efforts, new terms have sprung up in acknowledgement of the full range of roles children and adults play in fighting forces; CAFF and WAFF, referring to children/women associated (or formerly associated) with fighting forces, are two examples. A donor request for proposals for former-soldier reintegration support in Liberia included these terms, making explicit an intention to fully include females and males who were not necessarily armed fighters. However, cash for weapons and other approaches perpetuate barriers. In advance planning there is often a failure to fully incorporate lessons from other experiences. Strong efforts are needed to creatively engage demobilizing males in gender discussions and actions, including those aimed at promoting their recovery and addressing their former, present or potential role as perpetrators of gender-based violence.

Reintegration approaches have become increasingly holistic; even young people not formerly with fighting forces are supported through DDR efforts. For example, support may be provided for schools that serve all young people rather than for individual child soldiers. Similarly, directing attention to particularly vulnerable girls while also acknowledging and addressing the needs of others, including at-risk boys, goes a long way towards answering the concerns of each while also minimizing the risk of creating additional gender divides.

Minimum standards for education in emergencies

Adolescent- and youth-focused education in emergencies has received little attention in the context of humanitarian efforts; however, action to address the educational rights of young people in conflict and post-conflict situations is gaining international momentum with the emergence of the new Minimum Standards for Education in Emergencies, Chronic Crises and Early Reconstruction (MSEE). The MSEE were developed by the Inter-Agency Network for Education in Emergencies, in which UNESCO, UNHCR, UNICEF, and various NGOs and individuals participate and seek to fulfil commitments to achieve education for all, with an emphasis on child and youth education.[48] Action to bridge gender divides and ensure equal access to education is central to the MSEE framework. MSEE implementation and monitoring present important opportunities to address youth- and gender-related education issues. Vigilance on the part of the MSEE Working

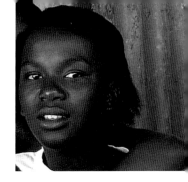

Group, which includes NGOs and United Nations agencies, is required to ensure that increased attention is given to the creation of appropriate educational opportunities for youth. Among other things, the Working Group should support the development of youth education field tools and pilot projects.

Global support is needed both to create opportunities for youth to complete primary and secondary education and to expand much-needed non-formal and vocational education. Some youth-focused education initiatives addressing the diverse learning needs of females and males, including demobilizing soldiers, offer examples of good practice and the opportunity to move forward. A major challenge is to expand life skills approaches in all programme action with youth so that young people can develop and employ values for living that help sustain peace and ensure the overall well-being of society.

Youth health and gender-based violence

The health sector continues to make progress in addressing issues of concern to youth, including those affected by armed conflict. Among many other initiatives, the Reproductive Health Response in Conflict Consortium (RHRC), consisting of research institutes and NGOs, has expanded its reproductive health programmes for young people.[49] A Minimum Initial Services Package has been developed along with other field tools to care for survivors of sexual violence, prevent the transmission of HIV, and reduce the incidence of maternal illness and death.

Despite these and other achievements, there are few mechanisms in place to ensure the consistent provision of available services to youth. Reproductive health programmes serving young people are often treated as subcomponents of health services for adults, and outreach to youth is limited. Data on participation in reproductive health programmes that serve a wide range of age groups are not regularly disaggregated, nor are good programme practices that have been shown to benefit youth routinely recorded or disseminated. Information about the different experiences of younger adolescents and older youth has not been fully assessed. Young people should be more fully involved in reproductive health programme planning, implementation and evaluation, with particular attention focused on access to services and the impact of initiatives on behavioural change.

Within the reproductive health context, advances have been made with regard to the prevention of HIV transmission and the care of people living with AIDS, with efforts extending to youth in many cases. Awareness-raising campaigns involving peer approaches, cultural events and media messages have been undertaken. Links with formal and non-formal education programmes have also been established to provide information about HIV/AIDS to in-school and out-of-school youth; such exposure represents an important component of life skills education. Some youth benefit from programmes focusing on the prevention of mother-to-child transmission and voluntary counselling and testing. Revised Guidelines for HIV/AIDS Interventions in Emergency Settings have been developed by the IASC[50] and are being disseminated and promoted. Efforts to address HIV/AIDS in emergency situations are still limited overall, however. Programmes that do exist should be more closely linked with gender-based violence services and increase their focus on youth. Youth-friendly approaches must be further developed and employed to ensure access for both younger and older youth.

Although achievements have not yet come close to meeting the enormous need, much substantive work has been done to expand innovative gender-based-violence programmes in humanitarian settings. Interventions range from education and awareness raising to psychosocial support and the provision of shelter, counselling, legal services, and medical and other care; again, youth are receiving a considerable amount of attention in many cases. A range of gender-based-violence training and other tools have been developed by the RHRC, and the IASC is in the process of finalizing its Guidelines for Gender-based Violence Interventions in Humanitarian Settings, including action sheets for wide distribution and coordinated use. Generally speaking, however, gender-based-violence programmes require additional resources and expansion and should be linked more closely with youth-focused responses, including children's, psychosocial, and education programmes. Stronger links with reproductive health programmes, including HIV/AIDS prevention and services, should also be established. Additional work with boys and men is needed to increase their awareness about gender-based violence, address their gender-based-violence needs, and strengthen their sense of responsibility for ending gender-based violence and fostering gender equality.

Youth and the Millennium Development Goals

Young people are involved with, and have a major stake in, the achievement of all the Millennium Development Goals (MDGs). Indicators for their well-being are explicitly mentioned in relation to the Goals on achieving universal primary education; promoting gender equality and empowering women; combating the spread of HIV/AIDS, malaria and other diseases; and developing a global partnership for development.[51] The Ad Hoc Working Group for Youth and the MDGs, consisting of representatives from youth organizations, recommends targeted support for girls and young women in the implementation of Goal 3 (relating to gender equality and women's empowerment), with particular attention given to improving their access to education. It emphasizes that building the capacity of, and creating sustained partnerships with, young people are crucial strategies for achieving the MDGs that have not been fully recognized by the international community. The Working Group calls for explicit attention to the situation of youth affected by armed conflict. However, suggestions for action are limited to the reintegration of former "combatants", support for post-conflict youth livelihoods, and a call for increased resources to facilitate open dialogue between youth and women (Ad Hoc Working Group for Youth and the MDGs, 2004).

The situation of youth affected by armed conflict should constitute a core issue in plans, policies and actions aimed at achieving the MDGs, given the numbers of countries and young people affected by armed violence. Within this context, a holistic approach is needed to address the explicit gender dimensions of conflict, with a conscious move away from the limited focus on "combatants", who are often perceived as exclusively male. Efforts should not be restricted to post-conflict environments; urgent action is also needed during emergency and protracted conflict situations, when critical assistance may be provided to refugee and IDP populations. Education initiatives must go beyond universal primary education for eligible younger children; appropriate and relevant education opportunities must also be made available to youth. The ten-year review of the World Programme of Action for Youth in 2005 represents an important opportunity to explicitly recognize the importance of gender, youth and armed conflict to the achievement of the MDGs, and to identify youth and conflict as a priority area in international action aimed at addressing the needs of young people.

Both gender and youth analyses are needed to ensure that the root causes and outcomes of armed conflict are better understood and more effectively addressed. Together, such analyses reveal the complex age and gender dynamics that are too often overlooked or misinterpreted in policy and programme approaches to war-affected populations. They challenge stereotypical interpretations of male youth as perpetrators and female youth as victims of violence, and of adults as protectors and young people as protected. They expose the inadequacies of narrow approaches to the protection and care of women and children, in particular the failure to take into account the age-specific experiences and contributions of youth, and offer new, more holistic options for conflict prevention, survival and recovery that may be coupled with more targeted approaches.

Adolescent girls and young women are more likely than male youth and young children to suffer gender-based violence. Male youth are the main perpetrators of gender-based violence and participate in armed violence. While these general patterns indicate how armed conflict worsens gender and age divides, they do not tell the whole story. In the upheaval of war, both groups play multiple roles that frequently extend beyond traditional gender, age and other social norms. The roles of females as armed fighters and of males as victims of sexual and other violence and deprivation are often misunderstood or ignored. Failure to recognize the diverse gender and youth realities in conflict and post-conflict settings results in missed opportunities to address gender inequalities and youth divides at their source and to create new, durable solutions for young people and their societies.

Too often, groups leading humanitarian aid, conflict prevention, reconstruction and peacebuilding efforts perpetuate gender and age divisions by employing short-term and/or narrowly defined approaches to women's and children's protection and care. Targeted "women and girls" approaches are greatly needed but should be adapted to better reflect age and broader gender realities. Youth-focused approaches should be expanded, but gender perspectives and considerations must be more effectively and consistently incorporated. Otherwise, females will continue to be left out of programmes for former soldiers, and few health and counselling services will address the needs of males or their roles in promoting gender equality. If education initiatives remain exclusively focused on young children, many adolescents and youth will be unable to acquire the skills they need to earn a sustaining livelihood or ensure their protection and security, with distinct negative consequences for males and females. If women's groups and youth groups continue to work separately, there will be little opportunity to develop integrated approaches for overcoming gender and youth inequalities at structural and other levels.

Both gender- and age-specific approaches must be incorporated into policy and programme planning, implementation and evaluation in ways that generate systemic change and transform social institutions and practices that reinforce male and adult dominance. Solutions must be youth-informed and, whenever possible, youth-driven, building on opportunities for social change that emerge out of conflict. These efforts require sufficient funding and a strong commitment at international, regional, national and local levels and must integrated, involving all sectors and phases of conflict prevention, response, recovery and development.

In support of the many specific recommendations included in the chapter, the following overarching recommendations for global action are proposed:

- Meeting in October 2005, the United Nations General Assembly may wish to identify youth and armed conflict as a priority within the World Programme of Action for Youth. The need for a combined age and gender approach to addressing the situation of youth affected by armed conflict should be made explicit in recognition of the diverse roles and contributions of male and female youth in survival and recovery from armed conflict. International action with and for youth should not be predicated solely on stereotypical interpretations of young people as violent actors or peacebuilders. It is highly desirable to initiate a coordinated United Nations effort to develop action, implementation and reporting plans. Among other things, this initiative might coordinate the development of a comprehensive action framework to address the needs of youth affected by armed conflict, engaging Member States, donors, other policymakers, practitioners and local community members, including youth, in this process. The framework should encompass a strong gender component and draw from emerging good practices, and should aim to expand understanding of the diverse rationales for working with youth affected by armed conflict.

- United Nations agencies, Governments, research institutes and other humanitarian and development actors should ensure that data collected on communities affected by armed conflict are disaggregated by age and sex, and that dynamic changes in age and gender norms are taken into account in programme implementation and evaluation. Policy and programme initiatives should respond to the diversity of youth experiences revealed through these efforts and should facilitate youth involvement in planning, implementation and evaluation efforts.

- The international community should provide expanded resources to build the capacities and support the rights of both male and female youth affected by armed conflict, with efforts focused on action-oriented youth leadership development, appropriate and relevant education initiatives that extend from armed conflict through post-conflict and into development, reproductive health programmes that incorporate HIV/AIDS awareness-raising and service provision, and sustained social and economic development that builds on informal and semi-formal youth livelihoods. Improved coordination between humanitarian and development actors is required.

- Reports on progress in meeting international commitments to human development and the protection of human rights should be age- and gender-specific and should address the particular circumstances of conflict-affected regions. Work to achieve the MDGs, Education for All, and a World Fit for Children should include attention to young refugees, IDP and other youth affected by conflict. Poverty Reduction Strategy Papers and the UNDP *Human Development Report* should explicitly address conflict and post-conflict situations and age- and gender-specific circumstances within these contexts. Young people should be involved in these and other processes, including efforts to monitor and report on the implementation of United Nations Security Council resolutions on children and armed conflict; the protection of civilians; and women and peace and security.

- Youth- and gender-focused action plans should be developed for the implementation, monitoring and evaluation of all guidelines adopted for the protection and care of war-affected populations, including the MSEE, the IASC Revised Guidelines for HIV Interventions in Emergency Settings, and the IASC Guidelines on Gender-Based Violence Interventions in Humanitarian Settings. Programming tools should be developed and pilot projects implemented that are focused on youth protection and development in these and other areas.

- Youth capacities and leadership should be supported at all levels of decision-making and action across programming sectors to ensure that youth-informed and youth-driven solutions are developed and that young people's potential as critical actors in contributing to individual and community survival and recovery is maximized. Particular attention should be given to ensuring the provision of opportunities for girls and young women, to promoting cooperation between males and females to achieve gender equality, and to strengthening relationships between adults and young people. Youth, women's, and other organizations at the local, national and international levels should establish and strengthen partnerships with one another to advance youth rights, gender equality, and efforts to ensure peace, conflict-prevention and recovery. ●

[1] Throughout this chapter, the term "youth" is used to refer to both females and males who may be identified as children or adults according to legal or cultural norms. "Young people" is used synonymously with "youth". "Adolescent boys and young men" and "adolescent girls and young women" are also used interchangeably with "male youth" and "female youth", respectively, to explicitly identify a gender and age group.

[2] The Convention on the Rights of the Child (United Nations, 1989) is the most widely ratified international treaty in history, having been endorsed by all countries except Somalia and the United States. Added more recently were the Optional Protocol on the Sale of Children, Child Prostitution and Child Pornography and the Optional Protocol on the Involvement of Children in Armed Conflict (United Nations, 2002a). *The Impact of Armed Conflict on Children*, a report commissioned by the United Nations and compiled by Graça Machel, was presented to the General Assembly in 1996; a follow-up review entitled *The Impact of War on Children* was released in 2001.

[3] Adolescents and youth affected by armed conflict have led a number of studies in which they articulate their concerns and offer recommendations for action, including with regard to gender (Cooper, 2004; Lowicki, 2005).

[4] This is due, in part, to the success of the International Coalition to Stop the Use of Child Soldiers and the adoption of the Optional Protocol to the Convention on the Rights of the Child on the Involvement of Children in Armed Conflict (United Nations, 2002a).

[5] According to the Rome Statute, adopted by the International Criminal Court in 1998, crimes against humanity include torture, rape, sexual slavery, enforced prostitution, forced pregnancy, enforced sterilization or any other comparably grave acts of sexual violence that are committed as part of a systematic attack on civilian populations (United Nations, 1998).

[6] The same could be said about the gender-based concerns of elderly women. In many contexts, youth and older persons affected by armed conflict face similar forms of marginalization owing to their age and socially defined status and roles, which may have undergone tremendous upheaval in armed conflict.

[7] A report published by the Institute of Development Studies emphasizes that consideration of gender issues in armed conflict must extend beyond stereotypical perceptions of males as aggressors and females as victims, with recognition given to the fact that both males and females play diverse roles in conflict situations (El-Jack, 2003).

[8] The focus in this chapter is on youth and gender, though it is recognized that many other factors also influence the experiences of youth affected by armed conflict, including socio-economic status, area of residence, religious beliefs, and membership in a particular ethnic or religious group.

[9] Some gender specialists strongly advise against using the word "gender" to denote the biological "sex" of an individual, arguing that gender has more complex connotations involving socially constructed norms and practices. However, "gender" continues to be used by most people in both contexts. In this chapter, the term sex is used only in reference to biological differentiations between males and females.

[10] These characterizations are employed by the United Nations Children's Fund, United Nations Population Fund, World Health Organization, and a number of other United Nations entities. National youth policies often reflect very different definitions of youth; in some cases the period of youth is interpreted as extending well into the 30s, while in other cases the bridge with childhood is eliminated with the exclusion of all young people below the age of 18.

[11] Many definitions and interpretations of armed conflict exist and may be obtained from a number of different sources, a few of which include the Uppsala Conflict Data Programme (available from www.pcr.uu.se/research/ucdp/index.htm); Project Ploughshares, which published the *Armed Conflicts Report, 2004* (available from www.ploughshares.ca/); and the International Crisis Group (ICG), which publishes *CrisisWatch*. *CrisisWatch* identifies countries affected by conflict and crisis, indicates the status of these conflicts, and provides alerts regarding potential outbreaks of conflict. In March 2005, the ICG identified nearly 70 countries or territories as conflict-affected (International Crisis Group, 2005). For young people, especially females, violence associated with armed conflict may continue during lulls in the fighting or even long after the official cessation of hostilities; gender-based violence (including domestic violence), various forms of social deprivation and/or discrimination, and inequalities and injustice take a very heavy toll on young women's lives.

[12] Refugees are those who have fled their homes or habitual residences and in so doing have crossed an international border; internally displaced persons (IDP) are displaced within the borders of their own countries or places of habitual residence. Returnees are those returning to their homes, villages and/or countries following a period of displacement as refugees or IDP. (See the United Nations Convention Relating to the Status of Refugees and the United Nations Office for the Coordination of Humanitarian Affairs' Guiding Principles on Internal Displacement.)

[13] According to the Global IDP Project, there were approximately 25.3 million IDP in the world as at December 2004 (Norwegian Refugee Council, 2004). Other statistics indicate that at the start of 2004, the number of people of concern to the Office of the United Nations High Commissioner for Refugees was 17.1 million, broken down as follows: 9.7 million refugees (comprising 57 per cent of the total); 985,500 asylum-seekers (6 per cent); 1.1 million returned refugees (6 per cent); 4.4 million IDP (26 per cent); and 912,200 others (5 per cent) (United Nations High Commissioner for Refugees, 2004).

[14] It is estimated that approximately 17.9 per cent (or a total of 1.157 billion) of the world's 6.464 billion people are between the ages of 15 and 24. In the least developed countries, however, this group comprises an average of 20.4 per cent of the population. Globally, females represent 49.74 per cent and males 50.26 per cent of the population (United Nations, 2004d; 2004e).

[15] Globally, 46.1 per cent of the population is under the age of 25, and in the least developed countries, many of which are affected by armed conflict, the percentage jumps to 62.2 per cent (United Nations, 2004d; 2004e).

[16] As at 30 September 2004, there were 966,266 Afghan refugees in Pakistan (see Pagonis, 2005). For statistics on Pakistan's under-25 population, see *World Population Prospects: The 2004 Revision* and *World Urbanization Prospects: The 2003 Revision* (United Nations, 2004d; 2004e).

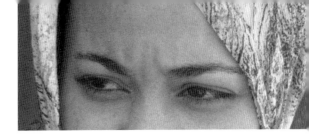

[17] Samuel Huntington (1996) is the author of *The Clash of Civilizations* and the *Remaking of World Order*.

[18] It should be noted that poverty, by itself, does not necessarily lead to the eruption of violence. Urdal (2004) argues that two additional factors—strong collective identity and the failure of political and economic structures to give groups opportunities to voice their demands peacefully-are needed to spur the expression of grievances over relative deprivation to the level of violence.

[19] Interview by the author with the Women's Commission for Refugee Women and Children, New York, July 2005.

[20] As aptly defined by Jeanne Ward in her book *If Not Now, When?*, "gender-based violence is an umbrella term for any harm that is perpetrated against a person's will, that has a negative impact on the physical or psychological health, development, and identity of the person; and that is the result of gendered power inequalities that exploit distinctions between males and females, among males and among females. Although not exclusive to women and girls, (gender-based violence) principally affects them across all cultures. Violence may be physical, sexual, psychological, economic or sociocultural." Many other forms of gender-based violence that may be worsened by armed conflict, including female infanticide, enforced sterilization and honour killings, are not considered within the scope of this chapter. Trafficking for sexual purposes is addressed in the present context, as it relates to refugee movements and participation in fighting forces.

[21] Even the involvement of a relatively small portion of the youth population in fighting forces has devastating consequences, as societies are plunged into wars from which it can take years to recover. It may also create an overall societal perception of youth (especially males) as violent and disruptive. This can create more barriers to opportunities for all youth. With their loss of education opportunities, youth may also be perceived as ignorant and not deserving of respect or opportunities to participate in community processes.

[22] See the Optional Protocol to the Convention on the Rights of the Child on the Involvement of Children in Armed Conflict (United Nations, 2002a). Article 1 prohibits children under the age of 18 from participating directly in hostilities, and article 2 bans the compulsory recruitment of children in this age group. Article 3 permits the voluntary recruitment of children under 18 years of age, with conditions.

[23] Yount and Balk (forthcoming) note that the World Health Organization (WHO) uses the term female genital mutilation, or FGM, to refer to all female genital practices, which it classifies into four groups. FGM is linked to female social identity and economic security in patriarchal societies, as those who undergo the procedure are allowed to marry and attain other privileges as adult women. The forms of FGM are diverse, and the practice is most prevalent in parts of Africa, Indonesia, Malaysia, the Arab Peninsula, and immigration countries. An estimated 130 million females have been affected, mainly in Africa, and 2 million females are at risk of FGM annually, according to WHO. The effects of FGM range from pain and incontinence to vaginal fistulae, infertility and even death. It also has wide-ranging psychosocial effects.

[24] The full privileges of womanhood, including eligibility for marriage, are achieved by undergoing FGM and entering a Secret Society.

[25] Yount and Balk (forthcoming) point out that according to some data, mean and median ages for FGM may be as low as 4 to 6 in some areas. If social and economic systems that support the practice are disrupted by war, FGM may be halted or delayed until adolescence. Refugee communities may have access to information on the dangers of FGM, including the transmission of HIV through the use of unclean instruments. In addition, women may have more access to information about women's experiences in other areas that are working to eliminate or develop safer alternatives to FGM while also ensuring the needed social outcomes.

[26] The case referred to was prosecuted under Kenya's 2002 Children's Act, as Kenya has jurisdiction over the refugee camps. The Act bans FGM.

[27] Other activities in this area have been undertaken by various United Nations agencies. In 1997, the United Nations Population Fund (UNFPA) appointed Ms. Waris Dirie as Goodwill Ambassador for the Elimination of Female Genital Mutilation, and the same year, the World Health Organization, United Nations Children's Fund and UNFPA published a joint statement on FGM, issuing an unqualified call for the elimination of this practice in all its forms (World Health Organization, 1997).

[28] Comparative adolescent-led research revealed that the early or forced marriage of adolescents was common in three diverse conflict and post-conflict settings, though the dynamics and thus the potential solutions were different (see Lowicki, 2004). Hundreds of thousands of adolescents and youth have become solely responsible for themselves and their siblings in communities affected by armed conflict, as their parents and other adult caretakers have died as a result of war or disease (including HIV/AIDS) or have gone missing.

[29] Telephone interview by the author with Carl Triplehorn, an education specialist with Save the Children in the United States, 18 July 2005.

[30] The Convention on the Rights of the Child guarantees basic education to children under the age of 18 and treats secondary education as a progressive right. Although international commitments to education for all have been made, humanitarian programmes focus mainly on the provision of formal primary education to primary-school-aged children. Older adolescents and youth have few opportunities to make up missed years or to find other appropriate and relevant education options. Support for the development of life skills is critical to all interventions with and for youth (see Sinclair, 2004; relevant information is also available at www.ineesite.org).

[31] See pages 15-17 for an analysis of gender and access to education in emergencies. Wider differences between male and female enrolment occur in specific countries and based on diverse refugee and cultural circumstances; see page 22 for details.

[32] Key reproductive health issues for youth in armed conflict include the following: early and unplanned pregnancy; complications in pregnancy and delivery; maternal mortality; STIs, including HIV/AIDS; unsafe abortions; gender-based violence, including rape, forced marriage, sexual enslavement and sexual exploitation; and genital mutilation. Girls under the age of 18 also face a high risk of complications during pregnancy and delivery. As the list indicates, females are more seriously affected than males in this context.

[33] Over 12 million young people have been orphaned by HIV/AIDS in Africa, leading to the creation of hundreds of thousands of youth-headed households, and many more such households have been created by armed conflict (Joint United Nations Programme on HIV/AIDS, 2004).

[34] Elements of this paragraph are taken from two unpublished documents: "Towards an IRC youth strategy" (Lowicki-Zucca, 2004b); and the "Draft integrated youth protection and development strategy" (Lowicki, 2005).

[35] When HIV/AIDS is prevalent in certain areas or among particular segments of society (including high-risk groups such as prostitutes, peacekeepers and injecting drug users) in the context of either generalized or concentrated epidemics, the risks are high that it will be transferred to vulnerable populations and communities in times of upheaval. Thus, communities newly exposed to people with the virus are newly at risk in armed conflict and post-conflict situations; the arrival of international peacekeepers is one example of such circumstances. At times, however, communities become increasingly isolated in armed conflict, which protects some youth from transmission. In addition, refugee youth may have more access to HIV/AIDS prevention information and care in armed conflict situations than previously (including access to voluntary counselling and testing, the prevention of mother-to-child transmission, post-exposure prophylaxis, and information-education-communication materials and services), and may also find new opportunities to participate in community activities relating to the prevention and treatment of HIV/AIDS. Another protective factor at times includes the cessation of FGM among female children and youth, as individuals in refugee situations often lack the resources or cultural support systems that ensure the continuation of this practice.

[36] Such participation has a number of benefits, both personal and societal. It helps youth develop communication and social skills, self-confidence, a sense of belonging and much more. As young people take the enthusiasm and ideas they develop further, it has exponential effects on their communities and societies (Lowicki, 2004).

[37] Interview with Mr. Amir Haxhikadrija, co-founder of the Kosovar Youth Council, London, May 2005 (unpublished).

[38] Women's Commission for Refugee Women and Children interviews with Ms. Akello Betty Openy and Mr. Ochora Emmanuel, co-founders of Gulu Youth for Action, Gulu, northern Uganda, December 2004 (unpublished).

[39] Areas covered in the adolescent-designed and adolescent-led research included Kosovo (2000), northern Uganda (2001) and Sierra Leone (2002).

[40] See the recommendations from the youth consultations under the section on armed conflict in the Youth Platform for Action (available from http://www.un.org/esa/gopher-data/conf/fwcw/pim/youth/youthpl.txt).

[41] The authors of this brochure are part of the Gender and Peacebuilding Working Group of the Canadian Peacebuilding Coordinating Committee, which undertook a study on the particular issues relating to girls and young women within the women and peace and security agendas; the study is slated for release in 2005.

[42] See the outcome document (Canada, no date). That same year, West African Ministers adopted the Accra Declaration and Plan of Action on War-Affected Children (Economic Community of West African States, 2000).

[43] See United Nations Security Council resolutions 1261, 1314, 1379, 1460 and 1539 (United Nations, 1999; 2000a; 2001b; 2003b; 2004c) (also available from http://www.un.org/docs/sc/index.html).

⁴⁴ The Youth Employment Network, established in accordance with relevant provisions in the Millennium Declaration, is a consortium of actors representing all sectors in support of youth employment. Heads of State at the Millennium Summit resolved to develop and implement strategies to support young people everywhere in finding decent and productive work (United Nations, 2003a).

⁴⁵ The Inter-Agency Standing Committee is comprised of both members (Food and Agriculture Organization of the United Nations, United Nations Office for the Coordination of Humanitarian Affairs, United Nations Development Programme, United Nations Population Fund, United Nations Children's Fund, Office of the United Nations High Commissioner for Refugees, World Food Programme, and World Health Organization) and standing invitees (International Committee of the Red Cross, International Council of Voluntary Agencies, International Federation of Red Cross and Red Crescent Societies, InterAction, International Organization for Migration, Steering Committee for Humanitarian Response, Representative of the Secretary-General on Internally Displaced Persons, Office of the United Nations High Commissioner for Human Rights, and World Bank) (see Inter-Agency Standing Committee, 2002).

⁴⁶ Frameworks for action with youth in crisis do exist in a variety of settings and may be applied to youth affected by armed conflict. However, a fundamental challenge exists in asserting key rationales for working with youth as a specific cohort, and more importantly, developing practical approaches that address their diverse realities.

⁴⁷ See note 245 in "Precious resources: participatory research study with adolescents and youth in Sierra Leone, April-July 2002" for analysis of the use of the term "combatant" to identify parties to the conflict in Sierra Leone and elsewhere and its relevance in planning and undertaking gender-aware disarmament, demobilization and reintegration efforts (Lowicki and Pillsbury, 2002).

⁴⁸ The Minimum Standards for Education in Emergencies, Chronic Crises and Early Reconstruction were developed by the Inter-Agency Network on Education in Emergencies through an extensive multi-year global consultative process (Norwegian Refugee Council, 2004).

⁴⁹ The Reproductive Health Response in Conflict Consortium consists of seven members. Four members-the American Refugee Committee, CARE, the International Rescue Committee, and Marie Stopes International-focus specifically on the provision of reproductive health services to refugees. Two members— Columbia University (Heilbrunn Center for Population and Family Health) and the JSI Research and Training Institute— are primarily involved in project research, staff training and technical assistance. The Women's Commission for Refugee Women and Children (the seventh member) plays a coordinating role for the Consortium and also lends technical assistance to NGOs providing health services. (See http://www.rhrc.org.)

⁵⁰ The Inter-Agency Standing Committee (IASC) was established in 1992 in response to General Assembly resolution 46/182 calling for strengthened coordination of humanitarian assistance. The Committee brings together United Nations and non-United Nations humanitarian partners. The primary role of the IASC is to formulate humanitarian policy to ensure coordinated and effective humanitarian response to complex emergency and natural disasters.

⁵¹ The Millennium Development Goals and targets are incorporated in the Millennium Declaration, signed by 189 countries, including 147 heads of State and Government, in September 2000 (available from http://www.un.org/millennium/declaration/ares552e.htm).

Bibliography

Ad Hoc Working Group for Youth and the MDGs (2004).Youth and the Millennium Development Goals: challenges and opportunities for implementation. Interim report of the Ad Hoc Working Group for Youth and the MDGs (available from http://www.unesco.org/wfeo/mdgyouthpaper.pdf).

Amnesty International (1998). Female genital mutilation: a human rights information pack. Section 7: United Nations initiatives (available from http://www.amnesty.org/ailib/intcam/femgen/fgm7.htm).

_____ (2000). Indonesia: a cycle of violence for Aceh's children (available from http://web.amnesty.org/library/index/ENGASA210592000).

_____ (2004a). Colombia: scarred bodies, hidden crimes; sexual violence against women in the armed conflict (available from http://web.amnesty.org/library/index/ENGAMR230402004).

_____ (2004b). Stop violence against women: Democratic Republic of the Congo-one woman's struggle for justice. AI Index: AFR 62/001/2004 (available from http://web.amnesty.org/library/index/ENGAFR620012004).

Bainvel, B. (1999). Youth participation: refugee camps in Kukes, Albania. New York: United Nations Children's Fund.

Bethke, L. (2004). *Global Survey on Education in Emergencies.* New York: Women's Commission for Refugee Women and Children.

Canada (no date). Caught in the Crossfire No More: A Framework for Commitment to War-Affected Children. Formal outcome document of the International Conference on War-Affected Children, held in Winnipeg, Canada, from 10 to 17 September 2000 (available from www.waraffectedchildren.gc.ca/crossfire-en.asp).

Coleman, I. (2005). Defending microfinance. Council on Foreign Relations (available from http://www.cfr.org/publication.html?id=7774).

Cooper, E. (2004). Empowerment through participatory action research: a case study of participatory action research with young refugees in Dagahaley Camp, Kenya. Master's thesis. Vancouver, Canada: University of British Columbia.

Economic Community of West African States (2000). Accra Declaration and Plan of Action on War-Affected Children in West Africa. Adopted at the Conference on War-Affected Children in West Africa, held in Accra, Ghana, on 27 and 28 April 2000.

Fleshman, M. (2005). Tough UN line on peacekeeper abuses. *Africa Renewal,* vol. 19, No. 1 (April).

Huntington, S.P. (1996). *The Clash of Civilizations and the Remaking of World Order.* New York: Simon & Schuster.

Inter-Agency Standing Committee (2002). Report of the Task Force on Protection from Sexual Exploitation and Abuse in Humanitarian Crises. 13 June.

_____ (2003). *Guidelines for HIV/AIDS Interventions in Emergency Settings.*

International Crisis Group (2005). CrisisWatch, No. 20 (1 April) (available from http://www.crisisgroup.org/home/index.cfm?id=2937&l=1#C1).

El-Jack, A. (2003). Gender and armed conflict: overview report. Brighton, United Kingdom: University of Sussex, Institute of Development Studies, BRIDGE (development-gender).

Joint United Nations Programme on HIV/AIDS (2004). *2004 Report on the Global AIDS Epidemic: 4th Global Report.* Geneva. UNAIDS/04.16E.

Kirk, J., and S. Taylor (2005). *Gender, Peace and Security Agendas: Where are Girls and Young Women?* Brochure, issued in March. Ottawa: Canadian Peacebuilding Coordinating Committee, Gender and Peacebuilding Working Group.

Lowicki, J. (2000). *Untapped Potential: Adolescents Affected by Armed Conflicts.* New York: Women's Commission for Refugee Women and Children.

_____ (2002). *Fending for Themselves: Afghan Refugee Children and Adolescents Working in Urban Pakistan.* Mission to Pakistan. New York: Women's Commission for Refugee Women and Children. January.

_____ (2004). *Youth Speak Out: New Voices on the Protection and Participation of Young People Affected by Armed Conflict.* New York: Women's Commission for Refugee Women and Children.

_____ (2005). Draft integrated youth protection and development strategy. Unpublished.

Lowicki-Zucca, J. (2004a). Interview with the International Rescue Committee's Gender-Based Violence Programme staff in Kono, Sierra Leone.

_____ (2004b). Towards an IRC youth strategy. Unpublished.

Lowicki, J., and M. Emry (2004). *No Safe Place to Call Home: Child and Adolescent Night Commuters in Northern Uganda.* New York: Women's Commission for Refugee Women and Children.

Lowicki, J., and A. Pillsbury (2002). Precious resources: participatory research study with adolescents and youth in Sierra Leone, April-July 2002. New York: Women's Commission for Refugee Women and Children.

Mandela, N. R. (1994). *The Illustrated Long Walk to Freedom: The Autobiography of Nelson Mandela.* Boston: Little, Brown & Co.

McKay, S., and D. Mazurana (2004). *Where Are The Girls?* Montreal: International Centre for Human Rights and Democratic Development.

Munala, J. (2003). Combating FGM in Kenya's refugee camps. *Human Rights Dialogue*, vol. 2, No. 10 (fall). Issue on violence against women. New York: Carnegie Council on Ethics and International Affairs (available from http://www.carnegiecouncil.org).

Newman, J. (2004). Voices out of conflict: young people affected by forced migration and political crisis: post-conference report, Cumberland Lodge, April 2004.

Norwegian Refugee Council (2004). IDP estimates. Global IDP Project: Monitoring Internal Displacement Worldwide (available from http://www.idpproject.org/statistics.htm).

Organization for Security and Co-operation in Europe (1999). Kosovo/Kosova — as seen, as told: an analysis of the human rights findings of the OSCE Kosovo Verification Mission, October 1998 to June 1999. Vienna: OSCE Office for Democratic Institutions and Human Rights.

Pagonis, J. (2005). Pakistani Afghan refugees suffer from bad weather. UNHCR Briefing Notes. Press briefing held on 8 March in Geneva (available from http://www.unhcr.ch/cgi-bin/texis/vtx/news/opendoc.htm?tbl=NEWS&id=422d89a84&page=news).

Parker, R.A., I. Lozano and L. Messner (1995). *Gender Relations Analysis: A Guide for Trainers.* Washington, D.C.: Save the Children.

Project Ploughshares (2004). *Armed Conflicts Report, 2004.* Ontario, Canada (available from http://test.ploughshares.ca/libraries/ACRText/ACR-TitlePageRev.htm).

Sinclair, M. (2004). *Learning to Live Together: Building Skills, Values and Attitudes for the Twenty-First Century.* Paris and Geneva: United Nations Educational, Scientific and Cultural Organization, International Bureau of Education.

Steinberger, M. (2001). So, are civilizations at war? Interview with Samuel P. Huntington. *The Observer* (21 October).

United Nations (1989). Convention on the Rights of the Child. A/RES/44/25. 20 November.

_____ (1991). Strengthening of the coordination of humanitarian emergency assistance of the United Nations. A/RES/46/182. 19 December.

_____ (1995). Fourth World Conference on Women: Platform for Action-Women and Armed Conflict (available from http://www.un.org/womenwatch/daw/beijing/platform/armed.htm).

_____ (1997). Women and sustainable development. Earth Summit+5: Special Session of the General Assembly to Review and Appraise the Implementation of Agenda 21, New York, 23-27 June (available from http://www.un.org/ecosocdev/geninfo/sustdev/womensus.htm).

_____ (1998). Rome Statute of the International Criminal Court (available from http://www.un.org/law/icc/statute/99_corr/cstatute.htm).

_____ (1999). Security Council resolution on children in armed conflict. S/RES/1261. 30 August.

_____ (2000a). Security Council resolution on the impact of armed conflict on children. S/RES/1314. 11 August.

_____ (2000b). Security Council resolution on women and peace and security. S/RES/1325. 31 October.

_____ (2001a). Promotion and protection of the rights of children: impact of armed conflict on children; note by the Secretary-General. A/51/306. 26 August.

_____ (2001b). Security Council resolution on the recruitment and use of children in armed conflict. S/RES/1379. 20 November.

_____ (2002a). Optional protocols to the Convention on the Rights of the Child on the involvement of children in armed conflict and on the sale of children, child prostitution and child pornography. Entered into force on 12 February 2002 and 18 January 2002, respectively; adopted by the United Nations General Assembly on 25 May 2000. A/RES/54/263. 26 June 2000.

_____ (2002b). A World Fit for Children: outcome document of the United Nations Special Session on Children, 8-10 May. A/RES/S-27/2. 11 October.

_____ (2003a). Promoting youth employment. General Assembly resolution 57/165 of 18 December 2002. A/RES/57/165. 16 January.

_____ (2003b). Security Council resolution on a call for halt to use of child soldiers. S/RES/1460. 30 January.

_____ (2003c). *World Population Prospects: The 2003 Revision* (available from http://esa.un.org/unpp/).

_____ (2004a). Report of the Secretary-General to the Security Council on the protection of civilians in armed conflict. S/2004/431. 28 May.

_____ (2004b). Report of the Secretary-General on women and peace and security. S/2004/814. 13 October.

_____ (2004c). Security Council resolution on children in armed conflict. S/RES/1539. 22 April.

_____ (2004d). *World Population Prospects: The 2004 Revision*. Population Database (available from http://esa.un.org/unpp/).

_____ (2004e). *World Urbanization Prospects: The 2003 Revision*. Sales No. E.04.XIII.6.

_____ (2005). Investigation by the Office of Internal Oversight Services into allegations of sexual exploitation and abuse in the United Nations Organization Mission in the Democratic Republic of the Congo. General Assembly report. A/59/661. 5 January.

United Nations Children's Fund (2005). Girls' education: promoting a culture of peace — a photo essay (available from http://www.unicef.org/girlseducation/14674_14675.html).

United Nations Development Programme (2003). World's top goals require women's empowerment. Message from UNDP Administrator Mark Malloch Brown on International Women's Day, 8 March (available from http://www.undp.org/dpa/statements/administ/2003/march/08mar03.html).

_____ (2005). Youth and violent conflict: society and development in crisis? A strategic review with a special focus on West Africa. New York: UNDP Bureau for Crisis Prevention and Recovery.

United Nations High Commissioner for Refugees (1999). *Reproductive Health in Refugee Situations: An Inter-Agency Field Manual*. Geneva.

_____ (2004). *Refugees by Numbers: 2004 Edition* (available from http://www.unhcr.ch/cgi-bin/texis/vtx/basics/opendoc.pdf?tbl=BASICS&id=416e3eb24).

Urdal, H. (2004) The devil in the demographics: the effect of youth bulges on domestic armed conflict, 1950-2000. Social Development Papers: Conflict Prevention & Reconstruction, Paper No. 14. Washington, D.C.: World Bank.

United States Agency for International Development (2004). *Youth & Conflict: A Toolkit for Intervention*. Washington, D.C.

Ward, J. (2002). *If Not Now, When? Addressing Gender-based Violence in Refugee, Internally Displaced and Post-Conflict Settings: A Global Overview*. The Reproductive Health for Refugees Consortium (now Reproductive Health Response in Conflict Consortium) (available from www.rhrc.org).

World Health Organization (1997). *Female Genital Mutilation: A Joint WHO/UNICEF/UNFPA Statement*. Geneva.

_____ (2000). *Reproductive Health during Conflict and Displacement: A Guide for Program Managers*. Chapter 17: understanding gender-based and sexual violence. WHO/RHR/00.13 (available from http://www.who.int/reproductivehealth/publications/RHR_00_13_RH_conflict_and_displacement).

_____ (2002). *World Report on Violence and Health*. Geneva.

Yount, K.M., and D.L. Balk (forthcoming). The health and social effects of female genital cutting: the evidence to date. Under review with Studies in Family Planning. Atlanta, Georgia: Emory University.

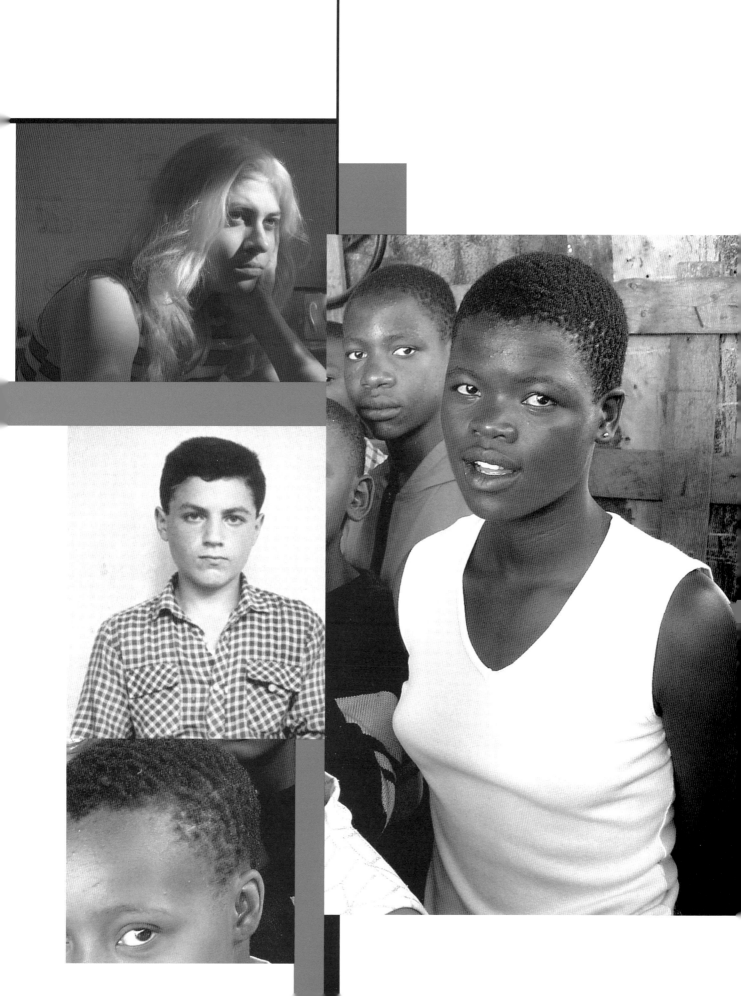

Litho in United Nations, New York
05 44737–October 2005–3000
ISBN 92-1-130244-7

United Nations publication
Sales No. E. 05 IV.6
ST/ESA/301